The Forgotten Home Apothecary Handbook:
400 Proven Remedies for Wellness, Vitality and Natural Healing

Author

Grace Thistle

Table of Contents

INTRODUCTION ---1
- The Origins of Natural Healing ---1
- Why Choose Natural Remedies? ---5
- How to Use This Book ---9

Quick Reference: Remedies by Ailment ---13

Digestive Health ---14
- Respiratory Support ---15
- Immune System Boosters ---16
- Pain Management ---17
- Skin and Hair Care ---18
- Stress and Emotional Well-Being ---19
- Women's Health ---20
- Men's Health ---21
- Children's Remedies ---22
- Elder Care ---23

The 400 Proven Remedies for Wellness and Vitality ---24

Digestive Health ---24
- Indigestion ---25
- Bloating ---26
- Constipation ---27
- Acid Reflux ---28
- Nausea ---29
- Diarrhea ---30
- Stomach Cramps ---32
- Flatulence ---33

Respiratory Support ---36
- Cough ---37

- Cold --- 38
- Nasal Congestion --- 39
- Sore Throat --- 40
- Bronchitis --- 41
- Wheezing --- 42
- Asthma Relief --- 44
- Mucus Reduction --- 45

Immune System Boosters --- 48
- Flu Prevention --- 49
- Energy Boost --- 50
- Cold and Flu Recovery --- 51
- Chronic Fatigue --- 52
- Antioxidant Support --- 53
- Immune Recovery --- 55
- Natural Antivirals --- 56

Pain Management --- 60
- Headaches --- 61
- Migraines --- 62
- Joint Pain --- 63
- Muscle Pain --- 64
- Back Pain --- 65
- Nerve Pain --- 67
- Arthritis --- 68
- General Pain Relief --- 69

Skin and Hair Care --- 72
- Acne --- 73
- Eczema --- 74
- Psoriasis --- 75

- Hair Loss — 76
- Dandruff — 77
- Skin Dryness — 79
- Dark Spots — 80
- Sunburn Relief — 81

Stress and Emotional Well-Being — 84
- Anxiety — 85
- Insomnia — 86
- Mood Swings — 87
- Burnout — 88
- Restlessness — 90
- Irritability — 91
- Depression — 92
- General Relaxation — 93

Women's Health — 96
- Menstrual Pain — 97
- PMS Symptoms — 98
- Menopause — 99
- Fertility Support — 100
- PCOS Relief — 101
- Vaginal Health — 103
- Breastfeeding Support — 104
- Hormone Balance — 105

Men's Health — 108
- Prostate Health — 109
- Stamina and Energy — 110
- Hair and Skin — 111
- Libido Support — 112

- Muscle Recovery — 114
- Heart Health — 115
- Stress and Performance — 116
- General Wellness — 117

Children's Remedies — 120
- Teething — 121
- Colic — 122
- Mild Fevers — 123
- Cough and Cold — 124
- Digestive Issues — 126
- Skin Irritations — 127
- Sleep Support — 128
- Immune Boosters — 129

Elder Care — 132
- Arthritis — 133
- Memory Support — 134
- Overall Vitality — 135
- Bone Health — 136
- Energy Support — 137
- Heart Health — 138
- Immunity — 140
- Skin and Wound Healing — 141

FAQs and Troubleshooting — 143
- Troubleshooting Common Issues — 147

Resources and Further Reading — 148

The Future of Natural Healing — 152

Closing Thoughts: A Message to the Reader — 156

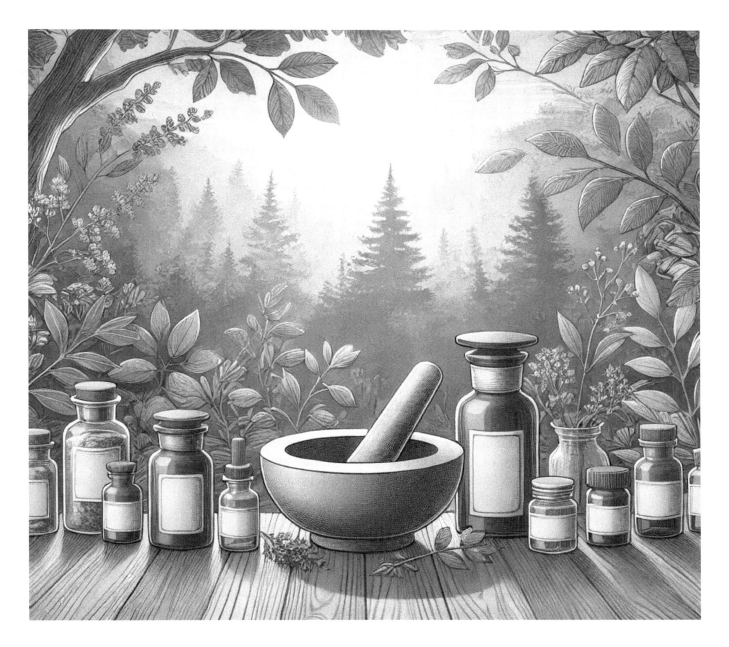

INTRODUCTION
The Origins of Natural Healing

Natural healing has deep roots in human history, stretching back thousands of years and spanning cultures across the globe. Long before the advent of synthetic pharmaceuticals, people relied on the gifts of nature—plants, minerals, and simple yet profound techniques—to treat illness, maintain wellness, and align themselves with the natural rhythms of the earth. These remedies, passed down through generations via oral traditions and ancient manuscripts, form the foundation of what we now call natural medicine.

The universality of natural healing lies in its ability to address human needs regardless of geography, era, or level of technological advancement. For millennia, civilizations thrived on the belief that health and nature are inseparable. The ancient Egyptians used honey for wound healing and embalming, while indigenous peoples of the Americas mastered the use of herbs to treat fever, pain, and digestive ailments. In South America, the Incas cultivated coca leaves for energy and altitude sickness, while the Chinese studied ginseng for vitality. These traditions, despite being separated by vast distances, often arrived at similar conclusions about certain plants' healing properties.

From the golden turmeric fields of India to the dense forests of North America, each culture developed its unique approach to healing based on the resources available to them and their understanding of the human body. While plants formed the cornerstone of natural healing, other elements like clay, minerals, and even animal products played a role in some traditions. For example, in medieval Europe, snail mucus was used for its skin-healing properties, while Ayurveda utilized cow's milk and ghee for internal and external healing.

Beyond treating illness, many healing traditions emphasized the importance of preventing disease. Practices like seasonal detoxes, balancing physical and mental health, and aligning one's daily habits with nature's rhythms were seen as essential to maintaining well-being. This preventive philosophy is still relevant today, particularly in the context of chronic diseases that modern medicine often struggles to address effectively.

Today, as the world faces increasing health challenges, the timeless wisdom of these traditions offers a valuable complement to modern medicine. The growing popularity of herbal supplements, essential oils, and natural therapies in the 21st century speaks to humanity's desire to reconnect with nature for healing. In particular, the sustainability of natural remedies has gained attention as an environmentally friendly alternative to synthetic drugs, which often carry heavy ecological costs.

Ayurveda: The Science of Life

Ayurveda, which translates to "the science of life," is one of the oldest known systems of medicine, originating in India over 3,000 years ago. At its core is the belief that health stems from a delicate balance between the body, mind, and spirit. Unlike modern medicine, which often targets symptoms, Ayurveda emphasizes prevention over cure, teaching individuals how to align their daily habits with the cycles of nature to maintain harmony.

The foundation of Ayurvedic medicine lies in the doshas:

- **Vata (air and space):** Governs movement, breathing, and circulation. People with a dominant Vata dosha may be prone to anxiety, dry skin, and digestive issues. Balancing Vata often involves warm, nourishing foods like soups and stews and calming practices such as yoga or meditation.

- **Pitta (fire and water):** Controls metabolism, digestion, and energy production. An imbalance can lead to inflammation, anger, or skin rashes. Cooling remedies like aloe vera juice, coconut water, and mint tea are often prescribed.

- **Kapha (earth and water):** Influences structure, immunity, and stability. Excess Kapha can result in sluggishness, weight gain, or respiratory problems. Spices like ginger, turmeric, and cinnamon are frequently recommended to invigorate and detoxify Kapha types.

Ayurvedic texts such as the **Charaka Samhita** and **Sushruta Samhita** provide detailed guidance on treating illnesses, balancing doshas, and using herbs effectively. These ancient manuscripts emphasize the integration of diet, lifestyle, and mental health to create a holistic approach to well-being.

Key Ayurvedic Practices:

1. **Herbal Formulations**:
- **Turmeric:** Anti-inflammatory and antioxidant properties for joint pain and skin conditions.
- **Ashwagandha:** Reduces stress and enhances energy levels.
- **Neem:** Potent antimicrobial for skincare and detoxification.
2. **Daily Routines (Dinacharya):** Practices like oil pulling, tongue scraping, and self-massage align daily habits with natural cycles.
3. **Panchakarma:** Detoxification treatments such as herbal enemas, therapeutic vomiting, and nasal cleansing.

Seasonal Adaptations:

Ayurveda emphasizes adapting one's habits to seasonal changes. For example:

- **Spring:** Bitter greens and light meals are recommended to cleanse Kapha buildup.
- **Summer:** Cooling fruits and drinks, such as watermelon and buttermilk, help balance Pitta.
- **Winter:** Warming spices like cinnamon, cardamom, and black pepper are used to pacify Vata.

By promoting a lifestyle of balance, mindfulness, and adaptability, Ayurveda offers practical solutions for maintaining health in today's fast-paced and often stressful world.

Traditional Chinese Medicine: Integrating Balance

Traditional Chinese Medicine (TCM) dates back more than 2,500 years and emphasizes the integration of balance, flow, and harmony in the body. Unlike Western medicine, which often isolates diseases to specific organs, TCM views health holistically. The philosophy centers on achieving equilibrium between **Yin and Yang**, opposite yet complementary forces, and promoting the smooth flow of **Qi**, the vital energy that courses through the body's meridians.

The Five Elements of TCM

The Five Elements—**Wood, Fire, Earth, Metal, and Water**—are the foundation of TCM's understanding of the body. These elements correspond to specific organs, emotions, and natural cycles:

- **Wood (Liver and Gallbladder):** Linked to creativity, renewal, and springtime. Imbalances can lead to frustration or anger.

- **Fire (Heart and Small Intestine):** Governs passion and vitality. Excess fire may cause anxiety or restlessness.
- **Earth (Spleen and Stomach):** Associated with nourishment and stability. Weakness in Earth may result in worry or fatigue.

Key TCM Practices for Wellness

1. **Acupuncture**: This practice involves inserting fine needles into specific meridian points to restore the flow of Qi.
2. **Herbal Medicine**: TCM utilizes a vast pharmacopeia of herbs tailored to individual needs. Popular herbs include:
- **Reishi Mushrooms:** Boost immunity and reduce inflammation.
- **Schisandra Berries:** Enhance focus and liver function.
- **Angelica Root:** Often called "female ginseng," it supports hormonal balance.
3. **Tai Chi and Qi Gong**: Combining breath control with slow, deliberate movements, these practices help regulate Qi and improve flexibility, strength, and mental clarity.

Western Herbalism: A Living Tradition

Western herbalism is deeply rooted in European traditions, enriched by the practices of Native American healers. It offers a blend of ancient remedies and modern science, presenting accessible solutions for everyday wellness.

Historical Roots of Western Herbalism

The Greek physician Hippocrates, often called the "Father of Medicine," emphasized treating the body with food and herbs rather than aggressive interventions. Medieval monks preserved and expanded on this knowledge, cultivating plants such as lavender, chamomile, and nettle for their therapeutic properties. Native American contributions, including the use of willow bark for pain relief and echinacea to boost immunity, further broadened the scope of Western herbalism.

Modern Applications

Today, herbalism is experiencing a resurgence as people seek sustainable alternatives to pharmaceuticals. Examples of widely used herbs include:

- **Turmeric:** A powerful anti-inflammatory and antioxidant.
- **Peppermint:** Effective for relieving digestive discomfort.
- **Valerian Root:** Known for promoting restful sleep and reducing anxiety.

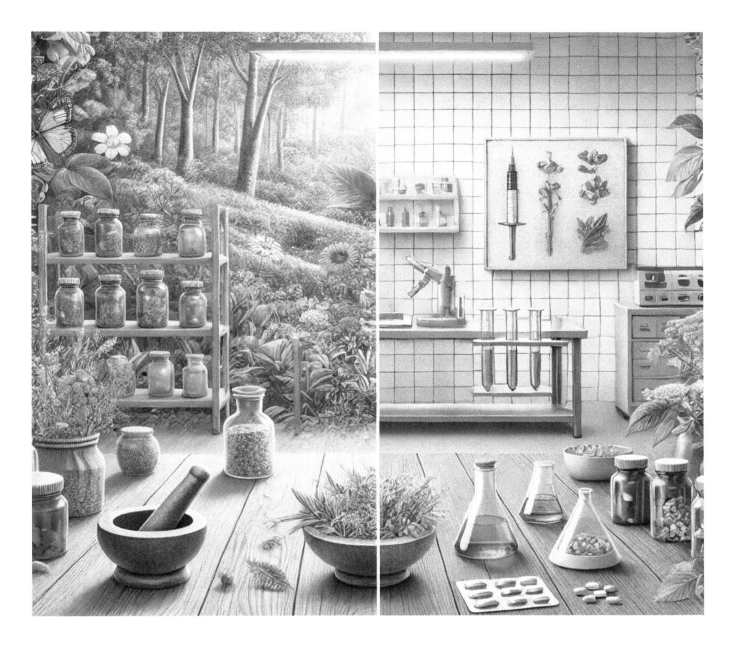

Why Choose Natural Remedies?

Natural remedies have been an integral part of human healing traditions for millennia. As interest in holistic health grows, people are rediscovering these age-old practices for their ability to promote wellness, prevent disease, and complement modern medical treatments. Unlike pharmaceuticals that often target specific symptoms, natural remedies aim to restore balance within the body, addressing both physical and emotional health.

The appeal of natural remedies lies in their accessibility, sustainability, and alignment with nature's rhythms. They empower individuals to take charge of their well-being while fostering a deeper connection to the environment and ancestral knowledge. In an era dominated by synthetic drugs and high healthcare costs, turning to nature offers not only a more sustainable solution but also a profound sense of harmony.

Benefits of Natural Remedies

1. Environmental Sustainability

Natural remedies are a reflection of nature's generosity, providing healing properties without the environmental toll of pharmaceutical production. The process of manufacturing modern medicines involves energy-intensive methods, chemical waste, and significant carbon emissions. For instance:

- Antibiotics and synthetic drugs can pollute waterways, harming aquatic life and contributing to antibiotic resistance in the environment.
- The extraction of raw materials for pharmaceuticals often involves deforestation or mining, further degrading ecosystems.

By contrast, cultivating medicinal plants such as **aloe vera**, **echinacea**, or **lavender** can actively support biodiversity and sustainable agriculture. Home-grown herbs reduce the reliance on mass production and long transportation chains, making healing more environmentally friendly.

Moreover, natural remedies are often biodegradable, leaving no harmful residues. This contrasts sharply with synthetic chemicals, which may persist in soil and water systems for years.

2. Minimal Side Effects

One of the most compelling reasons people choose natural remedies is their gentle impact on the body. While pharmaceuticals can be highly effective, they often come with side effects that range from mild discomfort to severe health complications. Examples include:

- Painkillers such as NSAIDs, which can cause stomach ulcers or kidney damage with prolonged use.
- Antibiotics, which may disrupt gut flora, leading to digestive issues or weakened immunity.

Natural alternatives often provide relief without these risks:

- **Peppermint oil** is a natural solution for headaches and indigestion, offering relief without dependency.
- **Turmeric**, known for its anti-inflammatory properties, is a safer long-term option compared to synthetic drugs like ibuprofen.

However, natural remedies are not entirely without risks. It's crucial to use them responsibly and with proper guidance, especially when combining them with conventional treatments.

3. Accessibility and Affordability

In many parts of the world, access to healthcare remains a significant challenge. Natural remedies offer an alternative that is both affordable and accessible. Unlike prescription drugs, which can cost hundreds of dollars, many remedies are available at a fraction of the price—or even free if grown at home.

For example:

- A simple infusion of **chamomile flowers** can help with insomnia or anxiety, costing only pennies per serving compared to pharmaceutical sleep aids.
- **Ginger root**, widely available and inexpensive, can treat nausea, improve circulation, and support digestion.

In addition to affordability, natural remedies empower individuals to take control of their health. Cultivating an herbal garden or learning basic preparation techniques fosters independence and reduces reliance on commercial healthcare systems. This self-sufficiency is particularly valuable in rural or underserved areas, where access to medical care may be limited.

4. Tradition and Innovation

The integration of ancient healing practices with modern research has led to remarkable advancements in natural medicine. Scientific studies now validate the efficacy of remedies that have been used for centuries. Examples include:

- **Ashwagandha**, a key herb in Ayurveda, which has been shown to reduce cortisol levels and combat stress.
- **Willow bark**, the precursor to aspirin, used historically by Native Americans and Europeans to alleviate pain and fever.

This blend of traditional knowledge and modern science not only enhances the credibility of natural remedies but also paves the way for new applications. For instance, researchers are exploring the potential of **psilocybin mushrooms** to treat depression and PTSD, demonstrating how natural substances can address even complex mental health conditions.

Comparison with Modern Medicine

1. Targeting Symptoms vs. Holistic Healing

Modern medicine often focuses on addressing symptoms, providing rapid relief for acute conditions. While this is invaluable in emergencies, it can sometimes overlook the root causes of chronic issues. Natural remedies, by contrast, aim to support the body's natural healing processes and restore balance.

For example:

- Instead of using antacids to neutralize stomach acid, remedies like **slippery elm tea** protect the stomach lining and address underlying inflammation.
- For anxiety, pharmaceuticals may temporarily mask symptoms, whereas a combination of **valerian root** and mindfulness practices can promote lasting emotional balance.

2. Personalized Care

Natural remedies inherently promote a personalized approach to healing. In systems like **Ayurveda** or **Traditional Chinese Medicine**, treatments are tailored to an individual's unique constitution, lifestyle, and environment. This contrasts with the standardized protocols of modern medicine, which often rely on generalized dosages and treatments.

Examples include:

- **Ayurveda**: By assessing doshas—Vata, Pitta, and Kapha—practitioners create customized plans to restore equilibrium.

- **Traditional Chinese Medicine**: The diagnosis of Qi imbalances leads to highly specific herbal prescriptions and lifestyle changes.

3. Cost Implications

The financial burden of healthcare in many countries, particularly in the United States, has led individuals to seek alternatives. Natural remedies often represent a fraction of the cost of conventional treatments. For instance:

- A course of prescription antibiotics can cost $50–$100, while a similar antibacterial effect can be achieved using **oregano oil** or **manuka honey** for much less.

- **Arnica gel**, used for bruises and muscle pain, is a budget-friendly alternative to commercial pain relief creams.

4. Complementary Use

Far from opposing modern medicine, natural remedies can be used to complement it. Combining these two approaches often yields better results, especially for chronic conditions or recovery after surgery.

For instance:

- **Acupuncture** and herbal teas can support cancer patients by reducing chemotherapy side effects such as nausea and fatigue.

- For joint pain, combining physical therapy with **turmeric capsules** or **ginger compresses** can enhance overall recovery.

Choosing natural remedies represents a shift toward a more balanced, sustainable, and personalized approach to health. While modern medicine remains a cornerstone of healthcare, natural remedies offer unique advantages that address gaps in the current system. By integrating the two, individuals can experience the best of both worlds: the precision and effectiveness of modern treatments combined with the holistic and preventive nature of natural healing.

Whether you're seeking relief from chronic pain, looking to boost your immune system, or simply wanting to reconnect with nature, natural remedies offer a path to wellness that is both time-tested and forward-looking. In embracing them, we honor the wisdom of the past while shaping a healthier and more sustainable future.

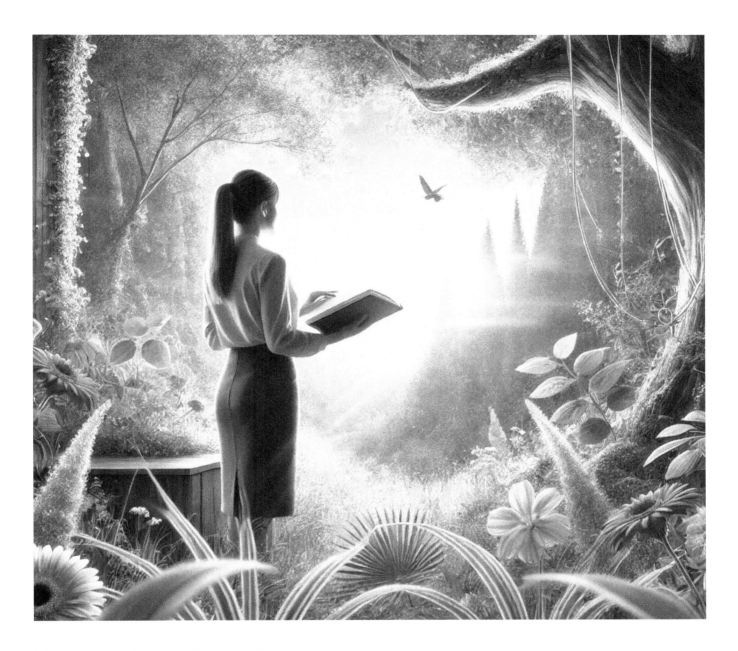

How to Use This Book

Welcome to **The Forgotten Home Apothecary Handbook**, a complete guide to natural healing and wellness. This book has been crafted to empower you with knowledge about remedies rooted in tradition and supported by nature. Whether you are new to herbal medicine or an experienced practitioner, this chapter will guide you on how to make the most of the content, turning information into practical action for your health and vitality.

Each chapter provides a window into the healing potential of nature, structured for easy navigation and tailored application. By following the instructions and tips in this section, you can unlock the full value of the remedies and make informed choices for your unique health journey.

Navigating the Book

Chapter Layout

The book is organized into chapters dedicated to specific health topics, such as Digestive Health, Respiratory Support, and Stress Management. Here's what to expect in each chapter:

1. **Introduction**: Provides an overview of the topic, discussing why it is significant and how natural remedies can address related issues.

2. **Remedy List**: This is the heart of each chapter, featuring detailed descriptions of remedies, their preparation methods, dosages, and expected outcomes. Remedies are listed starting with the most commonly used and widely accessible options.

3. **Conclusion**: Offers practical advice for integrating remedies into daily life, additional suggestions, or precautions to consider when using specific treatments.

This structure ensures a balance of foundational knowledge and actionable insights, allowing you to dive deeply into any health area that interests you.

Selecting Remedies

Matching Remedies to Ailments

A key feature of the book is the **Quick Reference: Remedies by Ailment** section, designed for fast problem-solving. Whether you're managing a chronic condition or addressing an acute symptom, this section points you directly to the relevant chapters and remedies.

For example:

- For insomnia, consult the **Stress and Emotional Well-Being** chapter, where you'll find options like chamomile tea, known for its calming properties, and valerian root tinctures for deeper relaxation.

- For persistent coughs or congestion, turn to the **Respiratory Support** chapter, which includes steam inhalation with eucalyptus oil and teas made with licorice root.

When selecting a remedy, consider factors such as the severity of your condition, the time required to prepare the remedy, and any known sensitivities you may have.

Customization and Safety

One of the strengths of natural remedies is their adaptability. You can tailor them to fit your needs by:

- Adjusting dosages according to your age, weight, and sensitivity levels.

- Choosing preparation methods that suit your preferences, such as teas, tinctures, or poultices.

- Combining remedies for enhanced effects; for example, pairing turmeric with black pepper to increase its bioavailability.

It's important to prioritize safety. Consult a healthcare professional if you:
- Have pre-existing conditions such as diabetes or cardiovascular issues.
- Are pregnant or breastfeeding.
- Are taking prescription medications, as interactions can sometimes occur.
- Experience persistent or worsening symptoms.

Tracking Your Progress

The Value of a Wellness Journal

Maintaining a wellness journal is one of the most effective ways to monitor how remedies work for you. By documenting your experiences, you can identify which treatments are most beneficial and fine-tune your approach. Include the following details in your journal:

- **Date**: Record when you began using a remedy.
- **Symptom**: Describe the issue you're addressing.
- **Remedy Used**: Note the preparation method, dosage, and frequency.
- **Results**: Observe and write down any changes, improvements, or side effects.

For example, if you're experimenting with remedies for anxiety, you might track how valerian root tinctures affect your sleep quality over a week or how lavender essential oil influences your mood during stressful days.

Experimentation and Gradual Progress

Natural remedies often involve a process of trial and observation. Begin with one remedy at a time to evaluate its effects before incorporating additional treatments. This approach reduces the risk of overwhelming your system or encountering unexpected interactions.

For example:

- If you're exploring digestive remedies, start with ginger tea for a week, noting its impact on bloating or nausea, before adding peppermint oil capsules to your routine.
- When managing stress, begin with aromatherapy using lavender essential oil. Once comfortable, integrate breathing exercises or a mindfulness practice alongside the remedy.

By taking a step-by-step approach, you build confidence and develop a deeper understanding of your body's responses.

Integrating Remedies into Daily Life

Building a Routine

Incorporating remedies into your daily routine can be simple and enjoyable. Start small by replacing a morning coffee with a herbal tea like green tea or nettle, which supports overall vitality. Over time, add practices such as evening baths infused with calming essential oils or weekly detoxes using recipes found in the Digestive Health chapter.

Combining with Modern Medicine

Natural remedies work well alongside conventional treatments. For example:

- If you're undergoing physical therapy for joint pain, supplementing with anti-inflammatory remedies like turmeric or ginger may enhance your recovery.
- During cold and flu season, you might use elderberry syrup to boost immunity while continuing to follow medical advice for symptomatic relief.

The integration of natural and modern approaches allows you to enjoy the benefits of both, addressing the root causes of health concerns while alleviating immediate discomfort.

This book is more than a collection of remedies—it's a guide to embracing a natural and intentional approach to well-being. By exploring the chapters, experimenting with remedies, and keeping track of your progress, you can take control of your health in a sustainable and personalized way. Approach each remedy with curiosity and patience, knowing that every step you take strengthens your connection to nature and your understanding of your body's needs.

Let this journey inspire you to rediscover the wisdom of nature, empowering you to build a lifestyle of vitality, balance, and resilience.

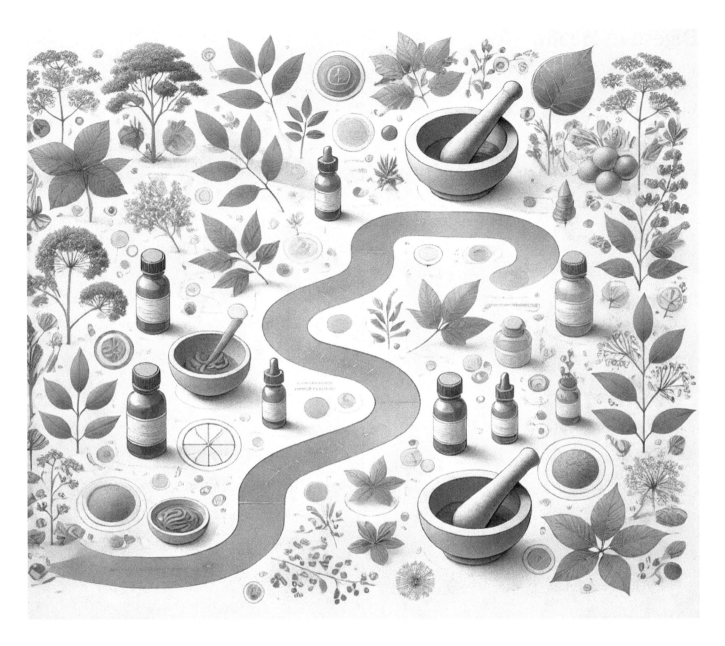

Quick Reference: Remedies by Ailment

This section is designed as a quick and easy-to-use index of remedies for a wide variety of health concerns. Whether you're dealing with a sudden symptom, planning preventive care, or managing chronic issues, you can use this guide to quickly find the remedies that address your needs.

Each category includes a total of 40 remedies, divided into specific ailments or conditions. Once you've identified the remedies of interest, turn to the corresponding chapters for detailed instructions on preparation, usage, and safety precautions.

Digestive Health

Indigestion

1. Ginger Tea
2. Apple Cider Vinegar
3. Peppermint Tea
4. Fennel Seeds
5. Baking Soda Solution

Bloating

6. Activated Charcoal
7. Peppermint Oil Capsules
8. Cumin Seed Tea
9. Chamomile Infusion
10. Caraway Seeds

Constipation

11. Psyllium Husk
12. Flaxseed
13. Aloe Vera Juice
14. Prune Juice
15. Magnesium Citrate

Acid Reflux

16. Slippery Elm Powder
17. Licorice Root Lozenges
18. Marshmallow Root Tea
19. Baking Soda Water
20. Cold Milk

Nausea

21. Ginger Chews
22. Lemon Water
23. Peppermint Lozenges
24. Clove Tea
25. Basil Leaves

Diarrhea

26. Blackberry Leaf Tea
27. Pomegranate Peel Infusion
28. Chamomile and Mint Tea
29. Fenugreek Seeds
30. Rice Water

Stomach Cramps

31. Warm Compress
32. Cinnamon Tea
33. Dill Seed Water
34. Anise Seed Infusion
35. Carom Seeds

Flatulence

36. Asafoetida Water
37. Ajwain Seeds
38. Dill Essential Oil
39. Ginger Capsules
40. Lemon Balm Tea

Respiratory Support

Cough

1. Honey and Lemon Tea
2. Thyme Infusion
3. Ginger Syrup
4. Marshmallow Root Tea
5. Licorice Root Lozenges

Cold

6. Elderberry Syrup
7. Garlic Broth
8. Echinacea Tea
9. Onion and Honey Syrup
10. Lemon Balm Tea

Nasal Congestion

11. Eucalyptus Steam Inhalation
12. Saline Nasal Spray
13. Peppermint Oil Diffusion
14. Chamomile Steam Therapy
15. Spicy Soup (with Chili and Ginger)

Sore Throat

16. Slippery Elm Lozenges
17. Salt Water Gargle
18. Honey and Cinnamon Paste
19. Clove Tea
20. Pomegranate Peel Decoction

Bronchitis

21. Turmeric Milk
22. Mullein Tea
23. Garlic and Honey Mixture
24. Ginger Compress
25. Fenugreek Tea

Wheezing

26. Basil Leaf Tea
27. Cinnamon and Honey Drink
28. Thyme Oil Massage
29. Peppermint Tea
30. Onion Syrup

Asthma Relief

31. Black Seed Oil Capsules
32. Ginger Tea with Honey
33. Tulsi (Holy Basil) Tea
34. Turmeric and Black Pepper Infusion
35. Licorice Root Tincture

Mucus Reduction

36. Lemon and Honey Hot Drink
37. Apple Cider Vinegar Rinse
38. Pineapple Juice (with Bromelain)
39. Hot Peppermint Tea
40. Warm Water with Salt

Immune System Boosters

Flu Prevention

1. Elderberry Syrup
2. Echinacea Capsules
3. Garlic Supplements
4. Turmeric Tea
5. Ginger Shots

Energy Boost

6. Ginseng Tea
7. Spirulina Smoothies
8. Bee Pollen Supplements
9. Maca Root Powder
10. Vitamin C Lozenges

Cold and Flu Recovery

11. Bone Broth
12. Lemon and Ginger Infusion
13. Honey and Garlic Syrup
14. Tulsi (Holy Basil) Decoction
15. Chamomile Tea

Chronic Fatigue

16. Ashwagandha Capsules
17. Rhodiola Rosea Tincture
18. Ginkgo Biloba Tea
19. Matcha Green Tea
20. Reishi Mushroom Powder

Antioxidant Support

21. Green Tea Capsules
22. Blueberry Smoothie
23. Pomegranate Juice
24. Nettle Infusion
25. Aloe Vera Water

Immune Recovery

26. Licorice Root Capsules
27. Zinc Supplements
28. Elderflower Infusion
29. Adaptogen Blends (Ashwagandha, Rhodiola)
30. Cod Liver Oil

Natural Antivirals

31. Oregano Oil Drops
32. Black Seed Oil Capsules
33. Lemon Balm Extract
34. Olive Leaf Tea
35. Garlic Oil Capsules

General Wellness

36. Probiotic Yogurt
37. Fermented Vegetables (e.g., Kimchi)
38. Wheatgrass Shots
39. Hibiscus Tea
40. Moringa Leaf Powder

Pain Management

Headaches

1. Peppermint Oil Massage
2. Feverfew Tea
3. Ginger Tea
4. Lavender Essential Oil Inhalation
5. Basil Leaf Infusion

Migraines

6. Butterbur Capsules
7. Magnesium Supplements
8. Cold Compress
9. Acupressure on Temple Points
10. Lemon Peel Paste

Joint Pain

11. Turmeric Paste
12. Ginger Compress
13. Epsom Salt Bath
14. Boswellia Capsules
15. Warm Mustard Oil Massage

Muscle Pain

16. Arnica Gel
17. Magnesium Oil Spray
18. Cayenne Pepper Cream
19. Chamomile Compress
20. Black Pepper Essential Oil Massage

Back Pain

21. Yoga Stretches (e.g., Cat-Cow Pose)
22. Warm Water Bottle Therapy
23. Devil's Claw Capsules
24. Turmeric Milk
25. Herbal Balm (Camphor and Eucalyptus)

Nerve Pain

26. St. John's Wort Oil
27. Passionflower Tea
28. Cold Packs for Acute Relief
29. Eucalyptus Oil Massage
30. Acupuncture Therapy

Arthritis

31. Ginger and Turmeric Tea
32. Warm Paraffin Wax Treatment
33. Omega-3 Supplements
34. Green Tea Extract Capsules
35. White Willow Bark Tea

General Pain Relief

36. Clove Oil for Topical Application
37. Valerian Root Capsules
38. Cabbage Leaf Compress
39. Evening Primrose Oil
40. Massage with Sesame Oil

Skin and Hair Care

Acne

1. Tea Tree Oil (Spot Treatment)
2. Witch Hazel Toner
3. Aloe Vera Gel Mask
4. Green Tea Ice Cubes
5. Neem Paste

Eczema

6. Oatmeal Bath
7. Calendula Cream
8. Coconut Oil Moisturizer
9. Vitamin E Oil
10. Chamomile Poultice

Psoriasis

11. Turmeric Cream
12. Fish Oil Supplements
13. Dead Sea Salt Bath
14. Licorice Extract Gel
15. Aloe Vera and Vitamin D Combo

Hair Loss

16. Rosemary Oil Scalp Massage
17. Onion Juice Treatment
18. Castor Oil Overnight Mask
19. Fenugreek Seed Paste
20. Amla Powder Hair Pack

Dandruff

21. Apple Cider Vinegar Rinse
22. Tea Tree Shampoo
23. Coconut Oil and Lemon Rub
24. Baking Soda Scrub
25. Aloe Vera and Neem Mix

Skin Dryness

26. Shea Butter Balm
27. Honey and Yogurt Mask
28. Avocado Oil Massage
29. Glycerin and Rose Water Spray
30. Olive Oil Moisturizer

Dark Spots

31. Potato Juice Treatment
32. Lemon and Honey Mask
33. Papaya Pulp Application
34. Sandalwood Paste
35. Vitamin C Serum

Sunburn Relief

36. Cold Milk Compress
37. Cucumber Gel
38. Aloe Vera Cooling Gel
39. Lavender Essential Oil Spray
40. Chamomile Infused Oil

Stress and Emotional Well-Being

Anxiety

1. Lavender Tea
2. Valerian Root Capsules
3. Chamomile Tea
4. Ashwagandha Powder
5. Passionflower Extract

Insomnia

6. Warm Milk with Nutmeg
7. Lavender Pillow Spray
8. Magnesium Supplements
9. Lemon Balm Tea
10. California Poppy Capsules

Mood Swings

11. St. John's Wort Capsules
12. Holy Basil Tea
13. Saffron Supplements
14. Bergamot Essential Oil Diffusion
15. Yoga and Pranayama Breathing

Burnout

16. Rhodiola Rosea Tincture
17. Adaptogenic Herb Mixes
18. Aromatherapy with Rosemary
19. Ginseng Tea for Energy Balance
20. Regular Walks in Nature

Restlessness

21. Epsom Salt Foot Bath
22. Peppermint Oil for Temple Massage
23. Warm Honey Lemon Drink
24. Acupressure on Calming Points
25. Guided Meditation Apps

Irritability

26. Cold Shower Therapy
27. Tulsi Tea
28. Cardamom Infused Water
29. Soft Music Therapy
30. Rose Tea

Depression

31. Saffron and Honey Mix
32. Regular Sunlight Exposure
33. Omega-3 Capsules
34. Journaling Practices
35. Ginkgo Biloba Tea

General Relaxation

36. Essential Oil Blends for Diffusion
37. Warm Herbal Baths
38. Relaxation Exercises (Progressive Muscle Relaxation)
39. Golden Milk (Turmeric and Milk)
40. Frankincense Incense Meditation

Women's Health

Menstrual Pain

1. Raspberry Leaf Tea
2. Hot Water Bottle Therapy
3. Ginger Tea with Honey
4. Evening Primrose Capsules
5. Fennel Seed Infusion

PMS Symptoms

6. Chasteberry Tincture
7. Magnesium and B6 Supplements
8. Black Cohosh Capsules
9. Peppermint Tea for Nausea
10. Lavender Oil Massage

Menopause

11. Sage Tea
12. Red Clover Supplements
13. Wild Yam Cream
14. Maca Root Powder
15. Flaxseed Smoothie

Fertility Support

16. Ashwagandha Root Powder
17. Shatavari Capsules
18. Royal Jelly Supplements
19. Dong Quai Tea
20. Adaptogenic Herb Mix

PCOS Relief

21. Spearmint Tea
22. Cinnamon Capsules
23. Omega-3 Fish Oil
24. Fenugreek Seed Water
25. Low-Glycemic Diet Support

Vaginal Health

26. Cranberry Juice for UTI Prevention
27. Probiotic Yogurt
28. Coconut Oil for Dryness Relief
29. Calendula Tea Wash
30. Aloe Vera Gel

Breastfeeding Support

31. Fenugreek Capsules
32. Blessed Thistle Tea
33. Warm Compress for Milk Flow
34. Fennel Seed Infusion
35. Oatmeal Diet

Hormone Balance

36. Evening Primrose Oil
37. Licorice Root Capsules
38. Holy Basil Infusion
39. Pumpkin Seed Mix
40. Green Smoothies with Maca

Men's Health

Prostate Health

1. Saw Palmetto Capsules
2. Pumpkin Seed Oil
3. Stinging Nettle Tea
4. Lycopene-Rich Foods (Tomatoes)
5. Flaxseed Oil

Stamina and Energy

6. Ginseng Root Tea
7. Beetroot Juice
8. Cordyceps Powder
9. Ashwagandha Tincture
10. Spirulina Smoothies

Hair and Skin

11. Rosemary Oil Scalp Massage
12. Aloe Vera for Skin Irritation
13. Olive Oil Moisturizer
14. Turmeric Capsules for Skin Health
15. Castor Oil for Beard Growth

Libido Support

16. Maca Root Powder
17. Horny Goat Weed Capsules
18. Tribulus Terrestris Supplements
19. Zinc Lozenges
20. Saffron Infusion

Muscle Recovery

21. Whey Protein Shakes
22. Tart Cherry Juice
23. Magnesium Spray for Sore Muscles
24. Epsom Salt Baths
25. Arnica Gel Application

Heart Health

26. Omega-3 Fish Oil Capsules
27. Hibiscus Tea
28. Garlic Extract Tablets
29. Coenzyme Q10 Supplements
30. Green Tea Infusion

Stress and Performance

31. Rhodiola Rosea Tea
32. Adaptogen Mix for Energy Recovery
33. Regular Cold Showers
34. Meditation with Lavender Oil
35. Regular Walks in Nature

General Wellness

36. Multivitamins with Minerals
37. Probiotic Supplements
38. Turmeric and Ginger Tea
39. Daily Bone Broth
40. Fermented Foods

Children's Remedies

Teething

1. Chamomile Tea Compress
2. Frozen Banana Teething Rings
3. Clove Oil Dilution for Gums
4. Silicone Teething Toys (Chilled)
5. Breastmilk Popsicles

Colic

6. Fennel Seed Water
7. Gripe Water (Homemade)
8. Warm Tummy Compress
9. Bicycle Leg Exercises
10. Baby Massage with Coconut Oil

Mild Fevers

11. Lukewarm Sponge Bath
12. Basil Tea for Fevers
13. Cooling Compress with Peppermint
14. Hydration with Coconut Water
15. Apple Cider Vinegar Wipes

Cough and Cold

16. Honey and Lemon Syrup (Over 1 Year)
17. Steam Inhalation with Eucalyptus (Supervised)
18. Ginger and Turmeric Milk
19. Saline Nasal Spray
20. Onion and Honey Cough Remedy

Digestive Issues

21. Chamomile Tea for Stomach Upset
22. Probiotic Drops
23. Warm Water with Ginger for Gas
24. Banana for Diarrhea Relief
25. Hydration with Electrolyte Drinks

Skin Irritations

26. Oatmeal Baths for Rashes
27. Calendula Cream for Irritation
28. Aloe Vera Gel for Mild Burns
29. Coconut Oil for Dry Skin
30. Cornstarch Powder for Chafing

Sleep Support

31. Lavender Pillow Mist
32. Bedtime Routine with Chamomile Tea
33. Gentle Massage with Almond Oil
34. Warm Milk with Honey (Over 1 Year)
35. White Noise Machine

Immune Boosters

36. Elderberry Syrup (Over 1 Year)
37. Vitamin C-Rich Fruits (e.g., Oranges)
38. Garlic Broth for Immunity
39. Probiotic Yogurt
40. Hydration with Herbal Infusions

Elder Care

Arthritis

1. Ginger and Turmeric Tea
2. Epsom Salt Foot Bath
3. Devil's Claw Capsules
4. Boswellia Extract
5. Warm Paraffin Wax

Memory Support

6. Ginkgo Biloba Capsules
7. Rosemary Oil Diffusion
8. Omega-3 Fish Oil
9. Vitamin D3 Supplements
10. Acupressure for Cognitive Function

Overall Vitality

11. Ashwagandha Powder in Milk
12. Bone Broth Soup
13. Herbal Green Smoothies
14. Spirulina Tablets
15. Bee Pollen

Bone Health

16. Calcium-Rich Foods (Sesame Seeds)
17. Vitamin K2 Supplements
18. Eggshell Calcium Powder
19. Nettle Tea for Minerals
20. Collagen Peptides

Energy Support

21. Maca Root Tea
22. Adaptogenic Herbs Mix
23. Morning Walks in Fresh Air
24. Holy Basil Leaf Infusion
25. Ginseng Tincture

Heart Health

26. Garlic Capsules
27. Hibiscus Tea Infusion
28. Pomegranate Juice
29. Hawthorn Berry Capsules
30. Coenzyme Q10

Immunity

31. Elderberry Syrup
32. Echinacea Tea
33. Reishi Mushroom Powder
34. Lemon and Honey Drink
35. Probiotic Supplements

Skin and Wound Healing

36. Calendula Ointment
37. Aloe Vera Gel for Burns
38. Comfrey Paste for Joint Pain
39. Manuka Honey for Wounds
40. Vitamin E Oil for Skin Repair

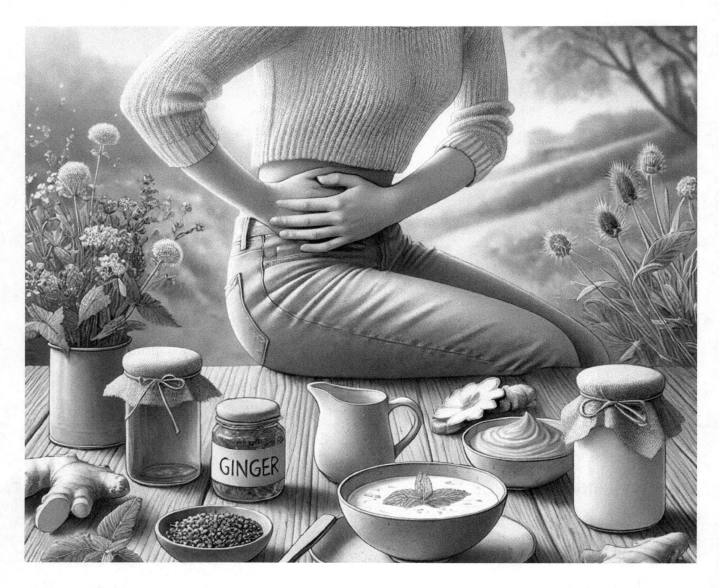

The 400 Proven Remedies for Wellness and Vitality
Digestive Health

Introduction

Digestive health plays a vital role in overall well-being. A well-functioning digestive system ensures optimal nutrient absorption, boosts immunity, and contributes to mental clarity. However, issues such as indigestion, bloating, or constipation can disrupt daily life and lead to discomfort.

This chapter explores 40 proven remedies that address common digestive ailments. These natural solutions focus on soothing discomfort, restoring balance, and supporting long-term digestive health. Whether it's the calming effects of herbal teas or the detoxifying power of activated charcoal, these remedies are designed to provide safe and effective relief.

Indigestion

1. **Ginger Tea**
   - **Ingredients**: 1 teaspoon of grated ginger, 1 cup of hot water
   - **Preparation**: Steep grated ginger in hot water for 10 minutes. Strain and drink warm.
   - **Why it Works**: Ginger aids digestion by stimulating gastric motility and reducing bloating.
   - **Pro Tip**: Add a dash of lemon juice or honey for enhanced flavor and additional soothing benefits.

2. **Apple Cider Vinegar**
   - **Ingredients**: 1 tablespoon of apple cider vinegar, 1 cup of warm water
   - **Use**: Mix apple cider vinegar with warm water and drink before meals.
   - **Why it Works**: Restores stomach acid levels and improves digestion, especially for protein-rich meals.
   - **Caution**: Avoid overuse to prevent enamel erosion.

3. **Peppermint Tea**
   - **Ingredients**: 1 teaspoon of dried peppermint leaves, 1 cup of hot water
   - **Preparation**: Steep peppermint leaves in hot water for 5 minutes. Strain and drink warm.
   - **Why it Works**: Peppermint relaxes the stomach muscles and alleviates indigestion.
   - **Tip**: Avoid if you suffer from acid reflux, as peppermint can exacerbate symptoms.

4. **Fennel Seeds**
   - **Ingredients**: 1 teaspoon of fennel seeds
   - **Use**: Chew fennel seeds after meals or steep them in hot water for a soothing tea.
   - **Why it Works**: Fennel reduces bloating and enhances digestion by relaxing intestinal muscles.
   - **Pro Tip**: Carry a small pouch of fennel seeds for on-the-go relief.

5. **Baking Soda Solution**
   - **Ingredients**: 1/2 teaspoon of baking soda, 1 cup of water

- **Use**: Dissolve baking soda in water and drink immediately.
- **Why it Works**: Neutralizes stomach acid and relieves indigestion quickly.
- **Caution**: Use sparingly to avoid disrupting the body's natural pH balance.

Bloating

6. **Activated Charcoal**
   - **Ingredients**: Pre-made activated charcoal capsules
   - **Use**: Take one capsule with water after meals, following product instructions.
   - **Why it Works**: Absorbs gas-producing toxins in the digestive system, reducing bloating.
   - **Caution**: Consult a doctor if you're on medication, as charcoal may reduce absorption.

7. **Peppermint Oil Capsules**
   - **Ingredients**: Pre-made peppermint oil capsules
   - **Use**: Take one capsule with water as needed.
   - **Why it Works**: Relaxes the gastrointestinal muscles and alleviates gas-related bloating.
   - **Pro Tip**: Look for enteric-coated capsules to prevent reflux.

8. **Cumin Seed Tea**
   - **Ingredients**: 1 teaspoon of cumin seeds, 1 cup of hot water
   - **Preparation**: Steep cumin seeds in hot water for 10 minutes. Strain and drink.
   - **Why it Works**: Cumin reduces gas and stimulates digestive enzymes for better digestion.
   - **Tip**: Toast the seeds before brewing for a richer flavor.

9. **Chamomile Infusion**
   - **Ingredients**: 1 teaspoon of dried chamomile flowers, 1 cup of hot water
   - **Preparation**: Steep chamomile flowers in hot water for 5 minutes. Strain and drink warm.
   - **Why it Works**: Soothes the stomach and reduces inflammation, easing bloating.
   - **Pro Tip**: Pair with peppermint for an enhanced calming effect.

10. **Caraway Seeds**

    - **Ingredients**: 1 teaspoon of caraway seeds
    - **Use**: Chew after meals or steep in hot water for a caraway tea.
    - **Why it Works**: Caraway relieves gas and bloating by relaxing intestinal muscles.
    - **Tip**: Combine with fennel seeds for a stronger digestive tonic.

Constipation

11. **Psyllium Husk**

    - **Ingredients**: 1 tablespoon of psyllium husk, 1 cup of water or juice
    - **Use**: Mix psyllium husk into water or juice and drink immediately, followed by an additional glass of water.
    - **Why it Works**: Psyllium is a natural fiber that absorbs water, softens stools, and promotes bowel movement.
    - **Pro Tip**: Start with a smaller dose to allow your body to adjust to the increased fiber intake.

12. **Flaxseed**

    - **Ingredients**: 1 tablespoon of ground flaxseed, 1 cup of water, smoothie, or yogurt
    - **Use**: Add ground flaxseed to smoothies, water, or yogurt daily.
    - **Why it Works**: Flaxseed provides soluble and insoluble fiber, improving stool bulk and regularity.
    - **Tip**: Store ground flaxseed in the refrigerator to maintain freshness.

13. **Aloe Vera Juice**

    - **Ingredients**: Pre-made aloe vera juice
    - **Use**: Drink 1/4 cup of aloe vera juice in the morning on an empty stomach.
    - **Why it Works**: Aloe vera contains natural laxative compounds that stimulate bowel movements.
    - **Caution**: Avoid overuse to prevent dependency or diarrhea.

14. **Prune Juice**

- **Ingredients**: Pre-made prune juice or fresh prunes
- **Use**: Drink 1/2 cup of prune juice daily or eat 3-4 prunes as a snack.
- **Why it Works**: Prunes are rich in sorbitol, a natural sugar alcohol that softens stools and promotes bowel movements.
- **Pro Tip**: Warm the juice slightly for enhanced effectiveness.

15. **Magnesium Citrate**
    - **Ingredients**: Pre-made magnesium citrate supplement
    - **Use**: Take one dose as directed on the label, preferably before bedtime.
    - **Why it Works**: Magnesium citrate draws water into the intestines, softening stools and relieving constipation.
    - **Caution**: Avoid overuse to prevent dehydration or electrolyte imbalances.

Acid Reflux

16. **Slippery Elm Powder**
    - **Ingredients**: 1 teaspoon of slippery elm powder, 1 cup of warm water
    - **Preparation**: Mix slippery elm powder into warm water and drink before meals.
    - **Why it Works**: Coats the stomach lining, reducing irritation and acid reflux symptoms.
    - **Pro Tip**: Add honey for added soothing effects.

17. **Licorice Root Lozenges**
    - **Ingredients**: Pre-made licorice root lozenges (DGL - deglycyrrhizinated licorice)
    - **Use**: Suck on one lozenge 15 minutes before meals.
    - **Why it Works**: Licorice soothes the esophagus and reduces acid production without raising blood pressure.
    - **Caution**: Use DGL lozenges to avoid glycyrrhizin-related side effects.

18. **Marshmallow Root Tea**
    - **Ingredients**: 1 teaspoon of dried marshmallow root, 1 cup of hot water

- **Preparation**: Steep marshmallow root in hot water for 10 minutes. Strain and drink warm.
- **Why it Works**: Marshmallow root forms a protective layer on the esophagus, reducing discomfort.
- **Pro Tip**: Drink after meals to prevent acid reflux symptoms.

19. **Baking Soda Water**
    - **Ingredients**: 1/2 teaspoon of baking soda, 1 cup of water
    - **Use**: Dissolve baking soda in water and drink immediately for quick relief.
    - **Why it Works**: Neutralizes stomach acid, providing fast relief from heartburn.
    - **Caution**: Use sparingly to avoid disrupting natural stomach acid balance.

20. **Cold Milk**
    - **Ingredients**: 1 cup of cold milk
    - **Use**: Drink a small amount of cold milk when symptoms of acid reflux arise.
    - **Why it Works**: Cold milk soothes the esophagus and reduces acid production temporarily.
    - **Pro Tip**: Use non-fat or low-fat milk to avoid exacerbating symptoms.

Nausea

21. **Ginger Chews**
    - **Ingredients**: Pre-made ginger chews or crystallized ginger
    - **Use**: Suck on one ginger chew or nibble small pieces as needed.
    - **Why it Works**: Ginger calms the stomach by blocking receptors responsible for nausea and promoting gastric emptying.
    - **Pro Tip**: Keep a pack of ginger chews handy during travel to prevent motion sickness.

22. **Lemon Water**
    - **Ingredients**: Juice of 1/2 lemon, 1 cup of warm or room-temperature water
    - **Preparation**: Mix lemon juice with water and sip slowly.

- **Why it Works**: Lemon's natural acidity and refreshing aroma help settle the stomach and ease nausea.
- **Pro Tip**: Add a small amount of honey for added soothing effects.

23. Peppermint Lozenges

- **Ingredients**: Pre-made peppermint lozenges or candies
- **Use**: Suck on one lozenge as needed to reduce nausea symptoms.
- **Why it Works**: Peppermint relaxes the stomach muscles and reduces spasms, helping to alleviate queasiness.
- **Caution**: Avoid peppermint if acid reflux is present.

24. Clove Tea

- **Ingredients**: 1/4 teaspoon of ground cloves, 1 cup of hot water
- **Preparation**: Steep ground cloves in hot water for 5 minutes. Strain and drink warm.
- **Why it Works**: Clove has mild anesthetic properties that calm the stomach and reduce nausea.
- **Pro Tip**: Sip slowly for the best effect.

25. Basil Leaves

- **Ingredients**: 5-6 fresh basil leaves, 1 cup of hot water
- **Preparation**: Steep basil leaves in hot water for 7-10 minutes. Strain and drink warm.
- **Why it Works**: Basil has calming and carminative properties that ease nausea and improve digestion.
- **Tip**: Chew on fresh basil leaves if tea isn't an option.

Diarrhea

26. Blackberry Leaf Tea

- **Ingredients**: 1 teaspoon of dried blackberry leaves, 1 cup of hot water
- **Preparation**: Steep blackberry leaves in hot water for 10 minutes. Strain and drink.
- **Why it Works**: Blackberry leaves contain tannins that tighten intestinal walls, reducing diarrhea.

- **Pro Tip**: Drink after every loose bowel movement for effective relief.

27. **Pomegranate Peel Infusion**
    - **Ingredients**: Dried pomegranate peel, 1 cup of hot water
    - **Preparation**: Simmer pomegranate peel in water for 5 minutes. Strain and drink warm.
    - **Why it Works**: The peel contains astringent compounds that reduce intestinal inflammation and control diarrhea.
    - **Pro Tip**: Store extra infusion in the refrigerator for up to 24 hours.

28. **Chamomile and Mint Tea**
    - **Ingredients**: 1 teaspoon each of chamomile flowers and dried mint leaves, 1 cup of hot water
    - **Preparation**: Steep chamomile and mint together in hot water for 10 minutes. Strain and drink warm.
    - **Why it Works**: Chamomile soothes the stomach, while mint reduces cramps and bloating.
    - **Tip**: Sip slowly to avoid exacerbating symptoms.

29. **Fenugreek Seeds**
    - **Ingredients**: 1 teaspoon of fenugreek seeds, 1 cup of water
    - **Use**: Swallow seeds with water or mix into yogurt for a calming effect on the digestive tract.
    - **Why it Works**: Fenugreek seeds form a protective gel that soothes irritated intestinal walls.
    - **Pro Tip**: Use sparingly to prevent bloating.

30. **Rice Water**
    - **Ingredients**: 1/2 cup of white rice, 2 cups of water
    - **Preparation**: Boil rice in water until tender, strain the liquid, and cool before drinking.
    - **Why it Works**: Rice water provides starch that binds stools and soothes intestinal inflammation.
    - **Pro Tip**: Drink in small sips throughout the day for best results.

Stomach Cramps

31. Warm Compress

- **Ingredients**: A clean cloth or heating pad, warm water
- **Use**: Soak the cloth in warm water, wring it out, and place it on the stomach. Alternatively, use a heating pad for 10-15 minutes.
- **Why it Works**: Heat relaxes abdominal muscles, reducing spasms and alleviating pain.
- **Pro Tip**: Combine with deep breathing exercises for enhanced relief.

32. Cinnamon Tea

- **Ingredients**: 1/2 teaspoon of ground cinnamon, 1 cup of hot water
- **Preparation**: Steep cinnamon in hot water for 10 minutes. Strain and drink warm.
- **Why it Works**: Cinnamon reduces gas and relaxes the intestinal muscles, easing cramping.
- **Pro Tip**: Add a touch of honey for sweetness and additional soothing effects.

33. Dill Seed Water

- **Ingredients**: 1 teaspoon of dill seeds, 1 cup of water
- **Preparation**: Boil dill seeds in water for 5 minutes. Strain and let cool before drinking.
- **Why it Works**: Dill has carminative properties that relieve gas and reduce stomach discomfort.
- **Pro Tip**: Drink after meals to prevent cramping.

34. Anise Seed Infusion

- **Ingredients**: 1 teaspoon of anise seeds, 1 cup of hot water
- **Preparation**: Steep anise seeds in hot water for 10 minutes. Strain and drink warm.
- **Why it Works**: Anise soothes the digestive tract and alleviates cramps by relaxing muscles.
- **Tip**: Pair with a light snack to reduce nausea associated with cramping.

35. Carom Seeds

- **Ingredients**: 1/2 teaspoon of carom seeds, a pinch of salt, 1/2 cup of warm water

- **Use**: Chew the seeds with salt and follow with warm water.
- **Why it Works**: Carom seeds improve digestion and reduce cramping by stimulating gastric juices.
- **Pro Tip**: Use sparingly to avoid excessive heat in the body.

Flatulence

36. **Asafoetida Water**

    - **Ingredients**: A pinch of asafoetida (hing), 1 cup of warm water
    - **Preparation**: Dissolve asafoetida in warm water and drink.
    - **Why it Works**: Asafoetida has antispasmodic properties that reduce gas and bloating.
    - **Pro Tip**: Mix with a pinch of black salt for enhanced effectiveness.

37. **Ajwain Seeds**

    - **Ingredients**: 1 teaspoon of ajwain seeds, a pinch of salt
    - **Use**: Chew the seeds with salt after meals.
    - **Why it Works**: Ajwain promotes digestion and reduces gas by stimulating gastric enzymes.
    - **Tip**: Pair with warm water for faster relief.

38. **Dill Essential Oil**

    - **Ingredients**: 2 drops of dill essential oil, 1 teaspoon of carrier oil (e.g., coconut or olive oil)
    - **Use**: Mix the essential oil with the carrier oil and massage gently onto the abdomen.
    - **Why it Works**: Dill oil relaxes intestinal muscles, relieving flatulence and cramping.
    - **Pro Tip**: Use in circular motions for better absorption and relaxation.

39. **Ginger Capsules**

    - **Ingredients**: Pre-made ginger capsules
    - **Use**: Take one capsule with water after meals.
    - **Why it Works**: Ginger reduces intestinal spasms and helps release trapped gas.

- **Pro Tip**: Opt for standardized capsules to ensure consistent potency.

40. **Lemon Balm Tea**

    - **Ingredients**: 1 teaspoon of dried lemon balm leaves, 1 cup of hot water
    - **Preparation**: Steep lemon balm leaves in hot water for 10 minutes. Strain and drink warm.
    - **Why it Works**: Lemon balm calms the digestive tract and reduces bloating, cramping, and gas.
    - **Pro Tip**: Sip before bedtime to aid digestion and promote relaxation.

Digestive Health: Summary

This section offers 40 natural remedies to address common digestive issues like **indigestion**, **bloating**, **constipation**, and **flatulence**. Each remedy is crafted to provide relief while supporting overall digestive health.

Key Takeaways Include:

- **Indigestion Relief**: Remedies like **ginger tea** and **fennel seeds** soothe discomfort and improve digestion.

- **Cramp Reduction**: Options like **cinnamon tea** and **warm compresses** offer quick relief from abdominal spasms.

- **Flatulence Control**: Solutions such as **asafoetida water** and **ajwain seeds** effectively reduce gas and bloating.

Incorporating these remedies into daily routines ensures a healthier, more comfortable digestive system. Always consult a healthcare provider for persistent symptoms or severe conditions.

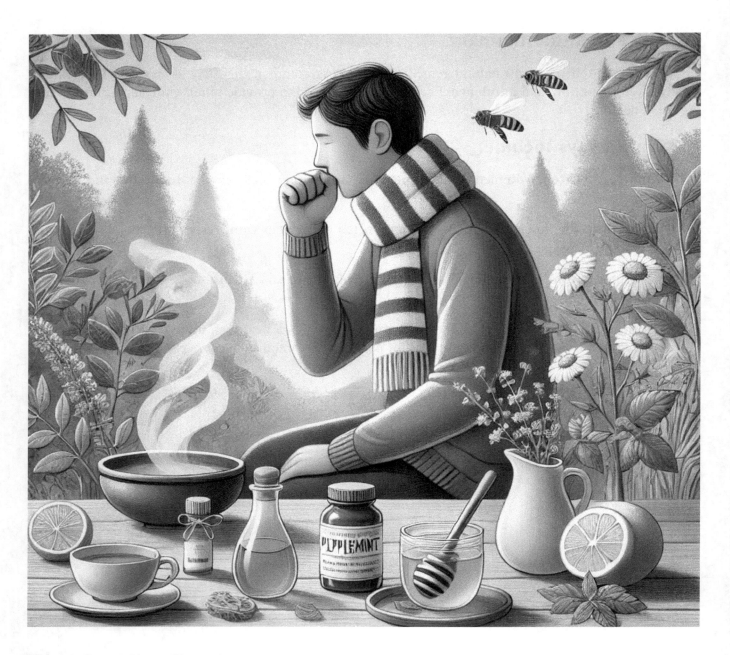

Respiratory Support

Introduction

Respiratory health is essential for maintaining energy, vitality, and overall well-being. Issues such as coughing, colds, and nasal congestion can significantly disrupt daily life, especially during seasonal changes. This chapter provides 40 natural remedies that offer safe and effective relief for respiratory concerns, focusing on soothing the airways, reducing inflammation, and supporting long-term respiratory health.

Whether it's the soothing effects of herbal teas or the anti-inflammatory power of turmeric milk, these remedies are designed to address specific respiratory issues with a holistic approach.

Cough

1. **Honey and Lemon Tea**

    - **Ingredients**: 1 tablespoon of honey, juice of 1/2 lemon, 1 cup of hot water

    - **Preparation**: Mix honey and lemon juice into hot water. Stir well and drink warm.

    - **Why it Works**: Honey coats the throat, reducing irritation, while lemon provides vitamin C and a refreshing flavor.

    - **Pro Tip**: Drink slowly to allow the honey to soothe the throat effectively.

2. **Thyme Infusion**

    - **Ingredients**: 1 teaspoon of dried thyme, 1 cup of hot water

    - **Preparation**: Steep thyme in hot water for 10 minutes. Strain and drink warm.

    - **Why it Works**: Thyme has antimicrobial properties and helps relax the respiratory muscles, reducing coughing fits.

    - **Tip**: Add a pinch of honey for extra throat relief.

3. **Ginger Syrup**

    - **Ingredients**: 1 tablespoon of grated ginger, 1 cup of water, 2 tablespoons of honey

    - **Preparation**: Simmer grated ginger in water for 10 minutes, strain, and mix the liquid with honey. Store in a jar and take 1 teaspoon as needed.

    - **Why it Works**: Ginger reduces inflammation in the airways and soothes persistent coughs.

    - **Pro Tip**: Keep refrigerated for up to 3 days for convenience.

4. **Marshmallow Root Tea**

    - **Ingredients**: 1 teaspoon of dried marshmallow root, 1 cup of hot water

    - **Preparation**: Steep marshmallow root in hot water for 10 minutes. Strain and drink warm.

    - **Why it Works**: Marshmallow root coats the throat and reduces irritation, calming dry or persistent coughs.

    - **Tip**: Combine with chamomile for a stronger calming effect.

5. **Licorice Root Lozenges**

- **Ingredients**: Pre-made licorice root lozenges
- **Use**: Suck on one lozenge as needed to soothe the throat.
- **Why it Works**: Licorice has anti-inflammatory properties that reduce throat swelling and calm coughing fits.
- **Caution**: Opt for deglycyrrhizinated licorice (DGL) lozenges to avoid blood pressure issues.

Cold

6. **Elderberry Syrup**
   - **Ingredients**: Pre-made elderberry syrup or homemade (elderberries, water, honey)
   - **Use**: Take 1 teaspoon daily during cold season or at the onset of symptoms.
   - **Why it Works**: Elderberry boosts immune function and reduces the duration of colds.
   - **Pro Tip**: Store homemade syrup in the refrigerator for up to 1 month.

7. **Garlic Broth**
   - **Ingredients**: 3 garlic cloves, 2 cups of water, a pinch of salt
   - **Preparation**: Simmer garlic in water for 10 minutes. Strain and drink warm.
   - **Why it Works**: Garlic has natural antimicrobial properties that fight cold viruses and boost immunity.
   - **Tip**: Add a squeeze of lemon for additional immune support.

8. **Echinacea Tea**
   - **Ingredients**: 1 teaspoon of dried echinacea, 1 cup of hot water
   - **Preparation**: Steep echinacea in hot water for 10 minutes. Strain and drink warm.
   - **Why it Works**: Echinacea enhances immune cell function, helping to reduce cold symptoms.
   - **Pro Tip**: Use at the first sign of a cold for maximum effectiveness.

9. **Onion and Honey Syrup**
   - **Ingredients**: 1 small onion, 2 tablespoons of honey
   - **Preparation**: Chop the onion and mix with honey. Let sit for 1 hour, strain, and take 1 teaspoon as needed.

- **Why it Works**: Onion's enzymes and honey's soothing properties reduce coughing and throat irritation.
- **Pro Tip**: Store in the refrigerator for up to 24 hours.

10. **Lemon Balm Tea**
    - **Ingredients**: 1 teaspoon of dried lemon balm leaves, 1 cup of hot water
    - **Preparation**: Steep lemon balm leaves in hot water for 5-7 minutes. Strain and drink warm.
    - **Why it Works**: Lemon balm calms the nerves and helps reduce cold-related stress and tension.
    - **Tip**: Drink before bedtime for improved sleep during a cold.

Nasal Congestion

11. **Eucalyptus Steam Inhalation**
    - **Ingredients**: 2-3 drops of eucalyptus essential oil, a bowl of hot water, a towel
    - **Use**: Add eucalyptus oil to a bowl of hot water. Cover your head with a towel and inhale the steam for 5-10 minutes.
    - **Why it Works**: Eucalyptus oil opens nasal passages, reduces inflammation, and helps clear mucus.
    - **Pro Tip**: Add a drop of peppermint oil for added decongestant effects.

12. **Saline Nasal Spray**
    - **Ingredients**: Pre-made saline nasal spray or homemade (1/4 teaspoon salt, 1 cup of distilled water)
    - **Use**: Administer 1-2 sprays into each nostril as needed.
    - **Why it Works**: Saline spray moisturizes nasal passages and flushes out allergens and irritants.
    - **Pro Tip**: Use before bedtime to reduce nighttime congestion.

13. **Peppermint Oil Diffusion**
    - **Ingredients**: 3-4 drops of peppermint essential oil, a diffuser
    - **Use**: Add peppermint oil to a diffuser and let it disperse in the room for 20-30 minutes.
    - **Why it Works**: Peppermint oil has menthol, which helps reduce nasal blockage and promotes easier breathing.

- **Tip**: Place the diffuser near your bed to support restful sleep.

14. **Chamomile Steam Therapy**
    - **Ingredients**: 1 teaspoon of dried chamomile flowers, a bowl of hot water
    - **Preparation**: Add chamomile flowers to hot water. Cover your head with a towel and inhale the steam for 5-10 minutes.
    - **Why it Works**: Chamomile soothes inflamed nasal tissues and reduces mucus buildup.
    - **Pro Tip**: Pair with a chamomile tea for a calming, double effect.

15. **Spicy Soup (with Chili and Ginger)**
    - **Ingredients**: 1 cup of chicken or vegetable broth, 1/2 teaspoon of chili flakes, 1 teaspoon of grated ginger
    - **Preparation**: Simmer broth with chili flakes and ginger for 5 minutes. Drink warm.
    - **Why it Works**: The spiciness of chili and the warming effect of ginger help clear nasal passages and improve mucus drainage.
    - **Tip**: Add garlic or turmeric for extra immune-boosting benefits.

Sore Throat

16. **Slippery Elm Lozenges**
    - **Ingredients**: Pre-made slippery elm lozenges
    - **Use**: Suck on one lozenge as needed to soothe the throat.
    - **Why it Works**: Slippery elm coats the throat, reducing irritation and pain.
    - **Pro Tip**: Look for lozenges with additional honey or licorice for enhanced soothing effects.

17. **Salt Water Gargle**
    - **Ingredients**: 1/2 teaspoon of salt, 1 cup of warm water
    - **Use**: Dissolve salt in warm water and gargle for 30 seconds. Repeat 2-3 times daily.
    - **Why it Works**: Salt water reduces swelling and kills bacteria in the throat, relieving soreness.
    - **Tip**: Add a pinch of turmeric for its antibacterial properties.

18. **Honey and Cinnamon Paste**
    - **Ingredients**: 1 teaspoon of honey, 1/4 teaspoon of cinnamon powder
    - **Preparation**: Mix honey and cinnamon into a smooth paste. Take small amounts throughout the day.
    - **Why it Works**: Honey soothes the throat, while cinnamon acts as a natural antibacterial agent.
    - **Pro Tip**: Use high-quality raw honey for maximum benefits.

19. **Clove Tea**
    - **Ingredients**: 1 teaspoon of whole cloves, 1 cup of hot water
    - **Preparation**: Steep cloves in hot water for 10 minutes. Strain and drink warm.
    - **Why it Works**: Clove has mild anesthetic properties that numb throat pain and reduce inflammation.
    - **Tip**: Add honey for sweetness and additional soothing properties.

20. **Pomegranate Peel Decoction**
    - **Ingredients**: 1 tablespoon of dried pomegranate peel, 1 cup of water
    - **Preparation**: Boil pomegranate peel in water for 5 minutes. Strain and let cool slightly before drinking.
    - **Why it Works**: Pomegranate peel is rich in antioxidants and tannins that soothe the throat and reduce inflammation.
    - **Pro Tip**: Store extra decoction in the fridge and reheat as needed.

Bronchitis

21. **Turmeric Milk**
    - **Ingredients**: 1/2 teaspoon of turmeric powder, 1 cup of warm milk
    - **Preparation**: Stir turmeric powder into warm milk and drink before bedtime.
    - **Why it Works**: Turmeric reduces inflammation in the bronchial tubes, easing breathing and discomfort.
    - **Pro Tip**: Add a pinch of black pepper to enhance curcumin absorption.

22. **Mullein Tea**
   - **Ingredients**: 1 teaspoon of dried mullein leaves, 1 cup of hot water
   - **Preparation**: Steep mullein leaves in hot water for 10 minutes. Strain and drink warm.
   - **Why it Works**: Mullein soothes the respiratory tract and helps clear mucus from the lungs.
   - **Pro Tip**: Combine with honey for added throat relief.

23. **Garlic and Honey Mixture**
   - **Ingredients**: 2 garlic cloves, 1 tablespoon of honey
   - **Preparation**: Crush garlic cloves and mix with honey. Let sit for 10 minutes before consuming.
   - **Why it Works**: Garlic fights respiratory infections, while honey soothes irritation.
   - **Tip**: Take once daily during acute bronchitis symptoms.

24. **Ginger Compress**
   - **Ingredients**: 2 tablespoons of grated ginger, a clean cloth, warm water
   - **Preparation**: Soak the cloth in warm water mixed with grated ginger. Apply to the chest for 15-20 minutes.
   - **Why it Works**: Ginger improves circulation and reduces chest congestion.
   - **Pro Tip**: Repeat twice daily for best results.

25. **Fenugreek Tea**
   - **Ingredients**: 1 teaspoon of fenugreek seeds, 1 cup of hot water
   - **Preparation**: Steep fenugreek seeds in hot water for 10 minutes. Strain and drink warm.
   - **Why it Works**: Fenugreek acts as a natural expectorant, helping to clear mucus from the lungs.
   - **Tip**: Add a pinch of turmeric for enhanced anti-inflammatory effects.

Wheezing

26. **Basil Leaf Tea**
   - **Ingredients**: 5-6 fresh basil leaves, 1 cup of hot water

- **Preparation**: Steep basil leaves in hot water for 7-10 minutes. Strain and drink warm.
- **Why it Works**: Basil reduces inflammation in the airways and eases wheezing.
- **Pro Tip**: Chew fresh basil leaves in case of sudden symptoms.

27. **Cinnamon and Honey Drink**
    - **Ingredients**: 1/4 teaspoon of cinnamon powder, 1 teaspoon of honey, 1 cup of warm water
    - **Preparation**: Mix cinnamon powder and honey into warm water and drink.
    - **Why it Works**: Cinnamon opens the airways, while honey soothes the throat and reduces irritation.
    - **Pro Tip**: Drink before bedtime for nighttime wheezing relief.

28. **Thyme Oil Massage**
    - **Ingredients**: 2 drops of thyme essential oil, 1 teaspoon of carrier oil (e.g., coconut or olive oil)
    - **Use**: Mix oils and massage gently onto the chest and back.
    - **Why it Works**: Thyme oil relaxes bronchial muscles and reduces wheezing.
    - **Pro Tip**: Use circular motions to improve absorption and circulation.

29. **Peppermint Tea**
    - **Ingredients**: 1 teaspoon of dried peppermint leaves, 1 cup of hot water
    - **Preparation**: Steep peppermint leaves in hot water for 5 minutes. Strain and drink warm.
    - **Why it Works**: Peppermint relaxes airway muscles and provides cooling relief.
    - **Tip**: Inhale the steam before drinking for added decongestant effects.

30. **Onion Syrup**
    - **Ingredients**: 1 medium onion, 2 tablespoons of honey
    - **Preparation**: Slice the onion, mix with honey, and let sit for 1 hour. Strain and take 1 teaspoon as needed.
    - **Why it Works**: Onion's anti-inflammatory properties and honey's soothing effects reduce wheezing and irritation.

- **Pro Tip**: Store in the refrigerator for up to 24 hours.

Asthma Relief

31. Black Seed Oil Capsules

- **Ingredients**: Pre-made black seed oil capsules
- **Use**: Take one capsule daily with water, following product instructions.
- **Why it Works**: Black seed oil reduces airway inflammation and supports respiratory function.
- **Pro Tip**: Combine with turmeric-based remedies for enhanced anti-inflammatory effects.

32. Ginger Tea with Honey

- **Ingredients**: 1 teaspoon of grated ginger, 1 cup of hot water, 1 teaspoon of honey
- **Preparation**: Steep ginger in hot water for 10 minutes. Strain and mix with honey. Drink warm.
- **Why it Works**: Ginger relaxes bronchial muscles and reduces airway constriction, while honey soothes irritation.
- **Pro Tip**: Drink twice daily during asthma flare-ups.

33. Tulsi (Holy Basil) Tea

- **Ingredients**: 5-6 fresh tulsi leaves, 1 cup of hot water
- **Preparation**: Steep tulsi leaves in hot water for 7-10 minutes. Strain and drink warm.
- **Why it Works**: Tulsi has anti-inflammatory and immune-boosting properties that help manage asthma symptoms.
- **Tip**: Chew fresh tulsi leaves for quick relief during mild attacks.

34. Turmeric and Black Pepper Infusion

- **Ingredients**: 1/2 teaspoon of turmeric powder, a pinch of black pepper, 1 cup of warm water
- **Preparation**: Mix turmeric and black pepper into warm water and drink daily.
- **Why it Works**: Turmeric reduces inflammation, and black pepper enhances curcumin absorption.
- **Pro Tip**: Drink on an empty stomach in the morning for optimal results.

35. **Licorice Root Tincture**
    - **Ingredients**: Pre-made licorice root tincture
    - **Use**: Add 10-15 drops of tincture to a glass of water or tea and drink daily.
    - **Why it Works**: Licorice soothes airways, reduces inflammation, and improves breathing.
    - **Caution**: Avoid overuse if you have high blood pressure; opt for deglycyrrhizinated licorice (DGL) tinctures.

Mucus Reduction

36. **Lemon and Honey Hot Drink**
    - **Ingredients**: Juice of 1/2 lemon, 1 teaspoon of honey, 1 cup of hot water
    - **Preparation**: Mix lemon juice and honey into hot water and drink warm.
    - **Why it Works**: Lemon helps break down mucus, and honey soothes the throat while reducing coughing.
    - **Pro Tip**: Drink in the morning to clear mucus accumulated overnight.

37. **Apple Cider Vinegar Rinse**
    - **Ingredients**: 1 tablespoon of apple cider vinegar, 1 cup of warm water
    - **Preparation**: Mix apple cider vinegar into warm water and drink slowly.
    - **Why it Works**: Apple cider vinegar thins mucus and promotes easier clearance.
    - **Caution**: Use sparingly to avoid disrupting stomach acid balance.

38. **Pineapple Juice (with Bromelain)**
    - **Ingredients**: 1 cup of fresh pineapple juice
    - **Use**: Drink 1 cup daily, preferably fresh.
    - **Why it Works**: Bromelain, an enzyme in pineapple, helps reduce mucus and inflammation in the respiratory tract.
    - **Pro Tip**: Combine with ginger for added anti-inflammatory benefits.

39. Hot Peppermint Tea

- **Ingredients**: 1 teaspoon of dried peppermint leaves, 1 cup of hot water
- **Preparation**: Steep peppermint leaves in hot water for 5 minutes. Strain and drink warm.
- **Why it Works**: Peppermint relaxes respiratory muscles and helps clear mucus.
- **Pro Tip**: Inhale the steam before drinking for enhanced effects.

40. Warm Water with Salt

- **Ingredients**: 1/2 teaspoon of salt, 1 cup of warm water
- **Use**: Gargle with the solution for 30 seconds, then spit out. Repeat as needed.
- **Why it Works**: Saltwater breaks down mucus and soothes the throat, reducing discomfort.
- **Pro Tip**: Gargle after meals to clear mucus effectively.

Respiratory Support: Summary

This chapter presented 40 natural remedies to address common respiratory concerns such as coughs, colds, asthma, and mucus buildup. These remedies are designed to provide effective relief while supporting long-term respiratory health.

Key Takeaways Include:

- **Asthma Management**: Options like **black seed oil capsules** and **turmeric infusions** reduce inflammation and improve breathing.

- **Mucus Reduction**: Remedies such as **pineapple juice** and **peppermint tea** help clear airways and promote easier breathing.

- **Overall Support**: Daily practices like **steam inhalation** and **herbal teas** ensure healthier airways and respiratory resilience.

Incorporating these remedies into daily routines can significantly improve respiratory health and quality of life.

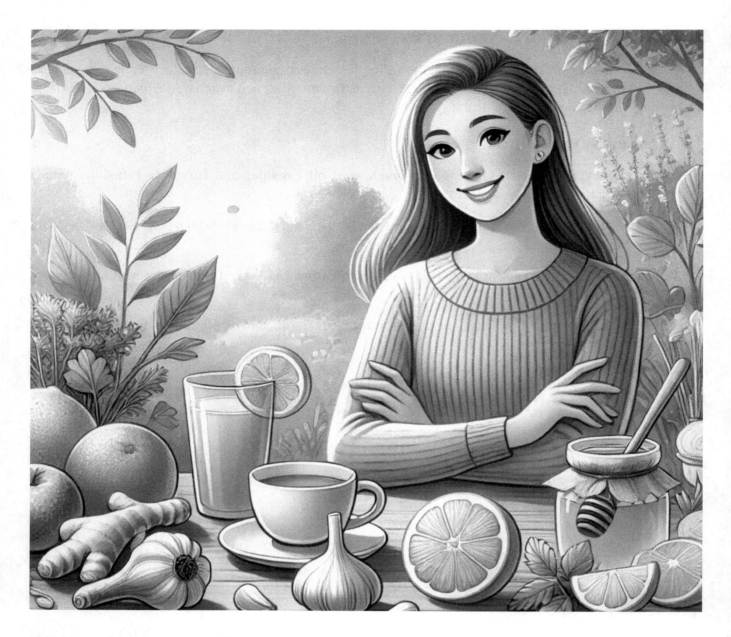

Immune System Boosters

Introduction

A strong immune system is the foundation of good health, helping the body defend against illnesses, recover quickly, and maintain vitality. This chapter provides 40 proven remedies to boost immunity, prevent infections, and support recovery from fatigue or illness. These natural solutions focus on enhancing immune function with antioxidants, adaptogens, and nutrient-rich foods, while providing effective strategies to maintain long-term wellness.

Flu Prevention

1. **Elderberry Syrup**

    - **Ingredients**: Pre-made elderberry syrup or homemade (elderberries, water, honey)
    - **Use**: Take 1 teaspoon daily during flu season or at the onset of symptoms.
    - **Why it Works**: Elderberries boost immune response and reduce the severity and duration of flu symptoms.
    - **Pro Tip**: Store homemade syrup in the refrigerator for up to 1 month for convenience.

2. **Echinacea Capsules**

    - **Ingredients**: Pre-made echinacea capsules
    - **Use**: Take one capsule daily as a preventive measure during flu season.
    - **Why it Works**: Echinacea enhances white blood cell activity, improving the body's ability to fight infections.
    - **Tip**: Use at the first sign of illness for maximum effectiveness.

3. **Garlic Supplements**

    - **Ingredients**: Pre-made garlic capsules or aged garlic extract
    - **Use**: Take one capsule daily with a meal.
    - **Why it Works**: Garlic has natural antimicrobial and immune-boosting properties that help prevent colds and flu.
    - **Pro Tip**: Include fresh garlic in meals for added immune support.

4. **Turmeric Tea**

    - **Ingredients**: 1/2 teaspoon of turmeric powder, 1 cup of hot water, optional: honey
    - **Preparation**: Mix turmeric powder into hot water and add honey if desired. Drink once daily.
    - **Why it Works**: Turmeric contains curcumin, which has anti-inflammatory and antioxidant properties that enhance immunity.
    - **Pro Tip**: Add a pinch of black pepper to increase curcumin absorption.

5. **Ginger Shots**

- **Ingredients**: 1 tablespoon of grated ginger, juice of 1/2 lemon, a pinch of cayenne pepper
- **Preparation**: Blend grated ginger and lemon juice with a splash of water. Strain and drink in a single shot.
- **Why it Works**: Ginger stimulates circulation, boosts immune response, and reduces inflammation.
- **Pro Tip**: Prepare a batch and store in small bottles for daily use.

Energy Boost

6. **Ginseng Tea**
   - **Ingredients**: 1 teaspoon of dried ginseng root slices, 1 cup of hot water
   - **Preparation**: Steep ginseng root in hot water for 10-15 minutes. Strain and drink warm.
   - **Why it Works**: Ginseng enhances energy and supports immune function by reducing fatigue.
   - **Pro Tip**: Drink in the morning for sustained energy throughout the day.

7. **Spirulina Smoothies**
   - **Ingredients**: 1 teaspoon of spirulina powder, 1 banana, 1 cup of almond milk
   - **Preparation**: Blend all ingredients until smooth and drink immediately.
   - **Why it Works**: Spirulina provides essential nutrients and antioxidants that boost energy and immunity.
   - **Pro Tip**: Add a handful of spinach for extra vitamins and minerals.

8. **Bee Pollen Supplements**
   - **Ingredients**: Pre-made bee pollen granules or capsules
   - **Use**: Take 1 teaspoon of granules or one capsule daily with a meal.
   - **Why it Works**: Bee pollen is packed with vitamins, amino acids, and enzymes that enhance stamina and immune response.
   - **Caution**: Avoid if allergic to bee products.

9. **Maca Root Powder**
   - **Ingredients**: 1 teaspoon of maca root powder, 1 cup of warm milk or water

- **Preparation**: Stir maca powder into the liquid and drink daily.
- **Why it Works**: Maca supports adrenal health, balancing energy and stress levels while boosting immunity.
- **Pro Tip**: Add to smoothies for a nutrient-packed breakfast option.

10. Vitamin C Lozenges

- **Ingredients**: Pre-made Vitamin C lozenges
- **Use**: Suck on one lozenge daily or as needed during flu season.
- **Why it Works**: Vitamin C strengthens the immune system and reduces the severity of colds.
- **Pro Tip**: Combine with zinc supplements for added immune-boosting effects.

Cold and Flu Recovery

11. Bone Broth

- **Ingredients**: Pre-made bone broth or homemade (simmered bones with vegetables and herbs)
- **Use**: Drink 1-2 cups daily during illness.
- **Why it Works**: Bone broth provides essential nutrients and minerals that support immune function and promote recovery.
- **Pro Tip**: Add garlic and ginger to enhance its immune-boosting properties.

12. Lemon and Ginger Infusion

- **Ingredients**: 1 tablespoon of grated ginger, juice of 1/2 lemon, 1 cup of hot water, optional: honey
- **Preparation**: Steep grated ginger in hot water for 10 minutes. Strain, add lemon juice, and sweeten with honey if desired.
- **Why it Works**: Ginger soothes inflammation, while lemon provides vitamin C to boost immunity.
- **Pro Tip**: Sip throughout the day to keep hydrated and reduce symptoms.

13. Honey and Garlic Syrup

- **Ingredients**: 2 cloves of garlic, 2 tablespoons of honey

- **Preparation**: Crush garlic cloves and mix with honey. Let sit for 1 hour. Take 1 teaspoon 2-3 times daily.
- **Why it Works**: Garlic's antimicrobial properties and honey's soothing effect help fight infection and reduce throat irritation.
- **Pro Tip**: Store in the refrigerator for up to 24 hours for repeated use.

14. Tulsi (Holy Basil) Decoction

- **Ingredients**: 5-6 fresh tulsi leaves, 2 cups of water, a pinch of black pepper
- **Preparation**: Boil tulsi leaves and black pepper in water until reduced to half. Strain and drink warm.
- **Why it Works**: Tulsi reduces mucus, boosts immunity, and relieves respiratory symptoms.
- **Pro Tip**: Add a teaspoon of honey for additional throat relief.

15. Chamomile Tea

- **Ingredients**: 1 teaspoon of dried chamomile flowers, 1 cup of hot water
- **Preparation**: Steep chamomile flowers in hot water for 10 minutes. Strain and drink warm.
- **Why it Works**: Chamomile soothes inflammation, relaxes muscles, and promotes restful sleep during illness.
- **Pro Tip**: Inhale the steam while steeping the tea to clear nasal passages.

Chronic Fatigue

16. Ashwagandha Capsules

- **Ingredients**: Pre-made ashwagandha capsules
- **Use**: Take one capsule daily with water, preferably in the evening.
- **Why it Works**: Ashwagandha supports adrenal health, reduces stress, and combats fatigue.
- **Pro Tip**: Combine with a bedtime routine for improved recovery from chronic fatigue.

17. Rhodiola Rosea Tincture

- **Ingredients**: Pre-made Rhodiola Rosea tincture

- **Use**: Take 10-15 drops diluted in water or tea once daily.
- **Why it Works**: Rhodiola improves energy levels and mental clarity while reducing fatigue caused by stress.
- **Pro Tip**: Use in the morning for sustained energy throughout the day.

18. **Ginkgo Biloba Tea**
    - **Ingredients**: 1 teaspoon of dried ginkgo leaves, 1 cup of hot water
    - **Preparation**: Steep ginkgo leaves in hot water for 10 minutes. Strain and drink warm.
    - **Why it Works**: Ginkgo biloba improves circulation and oxygen delivery, reducing symptoms of fatigue.
    - **Caution**: Avoid if taking blood-thinning medications.

19. **Matcha Green Tea**
    - **Ingredients**: 1 teaspoon of matcha powder, 1 cup of warm water or milk
    - **Preparation**: Whisk matcha powder into warm water or milk until frothy. Drink daily.
    - **Why it Works**: Matcha provides a steady energy boost and contains antioxidants that combat oxidative stress.
    - **Pro Tip**: Drink mid-morning for a sustained energy lift.

20. **Reishi Mushroom Powder**
    - **Ingredients**: 1/2 teaspoon of reishi mushroom powder, 1 cup of hot water
    - **Preparation**: Stir reishi powder into hot water and drink daily.
    - **Why it Works**: Reishi mushrooms reduce stress and support the immune system, helping combat chronic fatigue.
    - **Pro Tip**: Combine with a nightly relaxation ritual for improved recovery.

Antioxidant Support

21. **Green Tea Capsules**
    - **Ingredients**: Pre-made green tea extract capsules

- **Use**: Take one capsule daily with a meal.
- **Why it Works**: Green tea is rich in catechins, which combat oxidative stress and enhance immune function.
- **Pro Tip**: Combine with a morning cup of green tea for a double dose of antioxidants.

22. Blueberry Smoothie

- **Ingredients**: 1 cup of fresh or frozen blueberries, 1 banana, 1 cup of almond milk
- **Preparation**: Blend all ingredients until smooth. Drink immediately.
- **Why it Works**: Blueberries are loaded with anthocyanins, which protect cells from free radical damage.
- **Pro Tip**: Add a handful of spinach for extra vitamins and minerals.

23. Pomegranate Juice

- **Ingredients**: 1 cup of fresh pomegranate juice or seeds
- **Use**: Drink 1 cup daily, preferably fresh.
- **Why it Works**: Pomegranate is rich in antioxidants and polyphenols that support heart and immune health.
- **Pro Tip**: Choose unsweetened juice to maximize health benefits.

24. Nettle Infusion

- **Ingredients**: 1 teaspoon of dried nettle leaves, 1 cup of hot water
- **Preparation**: Steep nettle leaves in hot water for 10 minutes. Strain and drink warm.
- **Why it Works**: Nettle is a nutrient powerhouse, offering vitamins, minerals, and antioxidants that enhance immunity.
- **Pro Tip**: Pair with lemon for added flavor and vitamin C boost.

25. Aloe Vera Water

- **Ingredients**: 1/4 cup of aloe vera juice, 1 cup of water
- **Preparation**: Mix aloe vera juice with water and drink once daily.

- **Why it Works**: Aloe vera provides antioxidants and supports detoxification, improving overall health.
- **Pro Tip**: Use pure, organic aloe vera juice for maximum benefits.

Immune Recovery

26. **Licorice Root Capsules**
    - **Ingredients**: Pre-made licorice root capsules
    - **Use**: Take one capsule daily with water, following product instructions.
    - **Why it Works**: Licorice root soothes inflammation and supports immune recovery after illness.
    - **Caution**: Avoid prolonged use if you have high blood pressure; opt for deglycyrrhizinated licorice (DGL).

27. **Zinc Supplements**
    - **Ingredients**: Pre-made zinc tablets or lozenges
    - **Use**: Take one tablet or lozenge daily with food.
    - **Why it Works**: Zinc supports immune cell function and speeds up recovery from colds and flu.
    - **Pro Tip**: Combine with Vitamin C for enhanced immune-boosting effects.

28. **Elderflower Infusion**
    - **Ingredients**: 1 teaspoon of dried elderflowers, 1 cup of hot water
    - **Preparation**: Steep elderflowers in hot water for 10 minutes. Strain and drink warm.
    - **Why it Works**: Elderflower reduces inflammation and supports respiratory recovery after illness.
    - **Pro Tip**: Add honey to soothe a sore throat.

29. **Adaptogen Blends (Ashwagandha, Rhodiola)**
    - **Ingredients**: Equal parts ashwagandha and rhodiola powders, 1 cup of warm milk or water
    - **Preparation**: Mix powders into the liquid and drink daily.
    - **Why it Works**: Adaptogens reduce stress and promote immune resilience, aiding in recovery.

- **Pro Tip**: Use consistently for at least 4 weeks to see noticeable results.

30. Cod Liver Oil

- **Ingredients**: Pre-made cod liver oil capsules or liquid
- **Use**: Take one capsule or 1 teaspoon of liquid daily.
- **Why it Works**: Rich in vitamins A and D, cod liver oil supports immune recovery and bone health.
- **Pro Tip**: Choose a flavored version if using liquid to mask the fishy taste.

Natural Antivirals

31. Oregano Oil Drops

- **Ingredients**: Pre-made oregano oil drops, 1 cup of water or juice
- **Use**: Add 2-3 drops to water or juice and drink once daily.
- **Why it Works**: Oregano oil is rich in carvacrol and thymol, compounds with potent antiviral and antibacterial properties.
- **Pro Tip**: Use a dropper for precise dosing and avoid using directly on the tongue to prevent irritation.

32. Black Seed Oil Capsules

- **Ingredients**: Pre-made black seed oil capsules
- **Use**: Take one capsule daily with water.
- **Why it Works**: Black seed oil boosts immunity and fights viral infections with its active compound, thymoquinone.
- **Pro Tip**: Combine with a vitamin D supplement for added immune support.

33. Lemon Balm Extract

- **Ingredients**: Pre-made lemon balm tincture or extract
- **Use**: Take 10-15 drops diluted in water or tea once daily.
- **Why it Works**: Lemon balm contains rosmarinic acid, which combats viruses and reduces inflammation.

- **Pro Tip**: Use during cold sores or herpes outbreaks for faster healing.

34. **Olive Leaf Tea**
    - **Ingredients**: 1 teaspoon of dried olive leaves, 1 cup of hot water
    - **Preparation**: Steep olive leaves in hot water for 10 minutes. Strain and drink warm.
    - **Why it Works**: Olive leaves have antiviral compounds that inhibit virus replication and boost immune health.
    - **Pro Tip**: Add lemon and honey for enhanced flavor and additional soothing effects.

35. **Garlic Oil Capsules**
    - **Ingredients**: Pre-made garlic oil capsules
    - **Use**: Take one capsule daily with a meal.
    - **Why it Works**: Garlic oil contains allicin, which has strong antiviral and immune-boosting properties.
    - **Pro Tip**: Opt for odorless capsules if sensitive to garlic's strong scent.

General Wellness

36. **Probiotic Yogurt**
    - **Ingredients**: Organic, live-culture probiotic yogurt
    - **Use**: Consume 1/2 cup daily as a snack or part of a meal.
    - **Why it Works**: Probiotics support gut health, which is closely linked to overall immune function.
    - **Pro Tip**: Choose unsweetened yogurt to avoid added sugars that can weaken immunity.

37. **Fermented Vegetables (e.g., Kimchi)**
    - **Ingredients**: Pre-made fermented vegetables like kimchi or sauerkraut
    - **Use**: Add 2-3 tablespoons to meals daily.
    - **Why it Works**: Fermented foods are rich in probiotics and enzymes that improve digestion and immunity.

- **Pro Tip**: Incorporate into salads or as a side dish for added flavor and benefits.

38. Wheatgrass Shots

- **Ingredients**: 1 ounce of fresh wheatgrass juice or powder mixed in water
- **Use**: Drink one shot daily, preferably on an empty stomach.
- **Why it Works**: Wheatgrass provides chlorophyll, antioxidants, and essential nutrients that detoxify and strengthen the immune system.
- **Pro Tip**: Follow with a small glass of water to cleanse the palate.

39. Hibiscus Tea

- **Ingredients**: 1 teaspoon of dried hibiscus petals, 1 cup of hot water
- **Preparation**: Steep hibiscus petals in hot water for 10 minutes. Strain and drink warm.
- **Why it Works**: Hibiscus is packed with vitamin C and antioxidants that support immune health.
- **Pro Tip**: Serve cold as an iced tea for a refreshing alternative.

40. Moringa Leaf Powder

- **Ingredients**: 1 teaspoon of moringa leaf powder, 1 cup of warm water or smoothie
- **Preparation**: Mix moringa powder into water or a smoothie and drink daily.
- **Why it Works**: Moringa is a superfood with vitamins, minerals, and antioxidants that enhance immunity and energy.
- **Pro Tip**: Add to soups or stews for a savory boost.

Immune System Boosters: Summary

This chapter provided 40 remedies to strengthen immunity, combat viruses, and promote overall wellness. Each remedy harnesses the power of nature to protect the body and support recovery from illness.

Key Takeaways Include:

- **Antiviral Protection**: Options like **oregano oil** and **black seed oil** effectively combat viral infections.

- **Gut Health and Immunity**: Fermented foods such as **probiotic yogurt** and **kimchi** boost gut flora and enhance immune function.

- **Antioxidant Support**: Remedies like **hibiscus tea** and **blueberry smoothies** reduce oxidative stress and improve vitality.

Incorporating these remedies into daily routines can significantly enhance immune resilience and overall health.

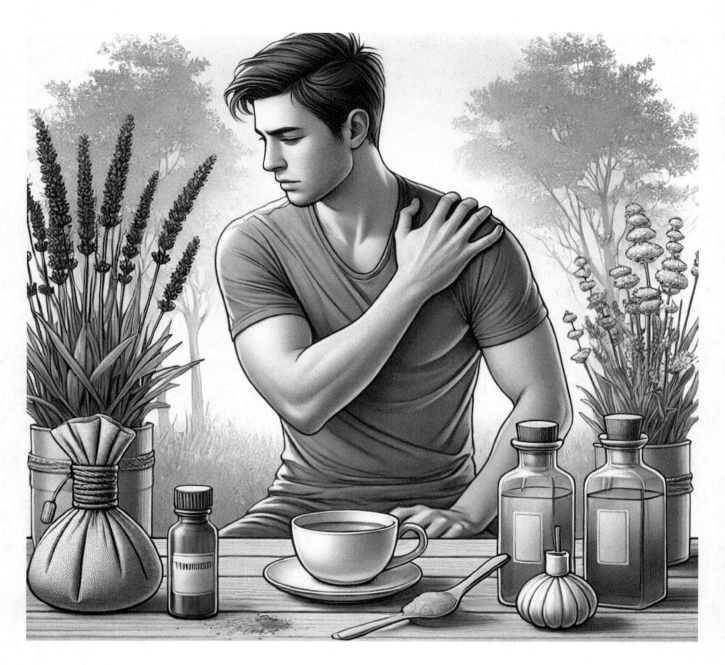

Pain Management

Introduction

Pain is a universal experience that can affect daily life, productivity, and emotional well-being. Whether it's a headache, joint discomfort, or muscle soreness, finding natural and effective ways to manage pain is essential. This chapter provides 40 remedies that address a variety of pain types, offering relief through herbs, essential oils, compresses, and lifestyle adjustments.

These remedies harness the power of nature to reduce inflammation, improve circulation, and promote relaxation, making them valuable tools for achieving comfort and balance.

Headaches

1. **Peppermint Oil Massage**

   - **Ingredients**: 2 drops of peppermint essential oil, 1 teaspoon of carrier oil (e.g., coconut or almond oil)
   - **Use**: Mix the oils and gently massage onto the temples and forehead.
   - **Why it Works**: Peppermint oil provides a cooling sensation and improves circulation, reducing headache pain.
   - **Pro Tip**: Inhale the scent during the massage for additional relief.

2. **Feverfew Tea**

   - **Ingredients**: 1 teaspoon of dried feverfew leaves, 1 cup of hot water
   - **Preparation**: Steep feverfew leaves in hot water for 10 minutes. Strain and drink warm.
   - **Why it Works**: Feverfew reduces inflammation and prevents the release of pain-inducing compounds in the brain.
   - **Caution**: Avoid if pregnant or breastfeeding.

3. **Ginger Tea**

   - **Ingredients**: 1 teaspoon of grated ginger, 1 cup of hot water
   - **Preparation**: Steep ginger in hot water for 10 minutes. Strain and drink warm.
   - **Why it Works**: Ginger reduces inflammation and relaxes blood vessels, alleviating headache symptoms.
   - **Pro Tip**: Add a slice of lemon for a refreshing twist.

4. **Lavender Essential Oil Inhalation**

   - **Ingredients**: 2-3 drops of lavender essential oil, a bowl of hot water
   - **Use**: Add lavender oil to hot water. Cover your head with a towel and inhale deeply for 5-10 minutes.
   - **Why it Works**: Lavender oil calms the nervous system and reduces tension, making it effective for stress-related headaches.
   - **Pro Tip**: Keep a small bottle of lavender oil handy for on-the-go inhalation.

5. **Basil Leaf Infusion**
    - **Ingredients**: 5-6 fresh basil leaves, 1 cup of hot water
    - **Preparation**: Steep basil leaves in hot water for 7-10 minutes. Strain and drink warm.
    - **Why it Works**: Basil acts as a muscle relaxant, relieving tension headaches caused by tight muscles.
    - **Pro Tip**: Chew a fresh basil leaf if tea isn't available.

Migraines

6. **Butterbur Capsules**
    - **Ingredients**: Pre-made butterbur capsules
    - **Use**: Take one capsule daily with water, following product instructions.
    - **Why it Works**: Butterbur reduces the frequency and severity of migraines by relaxing blood vessels in the brain.
    - **Caution**: Ensure the product is labeled "PA-free" to avoid toxic compounds.

7. **Magnesium Supplements**
    - **Ingredients**: Pre-made magnesium tablets
    - **Use**: Take one tablet daily with a meal.
    - **Why it Works**: Magnesium relaxes blood vessels and reduces the risk of migraines caused by magnesium deficiency.
    - **Pro Tip**: Combine with foods rich in magnesium, such as spinach or almonds, for added benefits.

8. **Cold Compress**
    - **Ingredients**: A clean cloth or ice pack, cold water
    - **Use**: Soak the cloth in cold water or use an ice pack wrapped in a towel. Apply to the forehead or back of the neck for 10-15 minutes.
    - **Why it Works**: Cold therapy constricts blood vessels, reducing pain and inflammation.
    - **Pro Tip**: Alternate with warm compresses to improve blood flow if the headache persists.

9. **Acupressure on Temple Points**

- **Use**: Use your fingertips to apply gentle pressure to the temples in a circular motion for 1-2 minutes.
- **Why it Works**: Acupressure releases tension and improves circulation, helping to relieve migraine pain.
- **Pro Tip**: Pair with deep breathing exercises for enhanced relaxation.

10. Lemon Peel Paste

- **Ingredients**: Peel of 1 lemon, a small amount of water
- **Preparation**: Grind the lemon peel into a paste using a blender or mortar and pestle. Apply to the temples for 10-15 minutes.
- **Why it Works**: Lemon peel's calming aroma and mild analgesic properties help reduce migraine intensity.
- **Pro Tip**: Use fresh lemon peels for maximum potency.

Joint Pain

11. Turmeric Paste

- **Ingredients**: 1 teaspoon of turmeric powder, a few drops of water
- **Preparation**: Mix turmeric powder with water to form a paste. Apply to the affected area and cover with a clean cloth for 15-20 minutes.
- **Why it Works**: Turmeric's curcumin reduces inflammation and eases joint stiffness.
- **Pro Tip**: Add a pinch of black pepper to the paste for enhanced absorption.

12. Ginger Compress

- **Ingredients**: 2 tablespoons of grated ginger, a clean cloth, warm water
- **Preparation**: Boil grated ginger in water for 5 minutes. Soak the cloth in the solution, wring it out, and apply to the joint for 15-20 minutes.
- **Why it Works**: Ginger improves circulation and reduces swelling around joints.
- **Pro Tip**: Repeat daily for ongoing relief.

13. Epsom Salt Bath

- **Ingredients**: 1-2 cups of Epsom salt, warm water
- **Preparation**: Dissolve Epsom salt in a warm bath and soak for 20-30 minutes.
- **Why it Works**: Magnesium in Epsom salt relaxes muscles and reduces joint inflammation.
- **Pro Tip**: Add a few drops of lavender oil for additional relaxation benefits.

14. **Boswellia Capsules**
    - **Ingredients**: Pre-made Boswellia (frankincense) capsules
    - **Use**: Take one capsule daily with water, following product instructions.
    - **Why it Works**: Boswellia reduces inflammation and supports cartilage health, improving joint mobility.
    - **Pro Tip**: Pair with turmeric supplements for a synergistic effect.

15. **Warm Mustard Oil Massage**
    - **Ingredients**: 2 tablespoons of mustard oil, 1 teaspoon of garlic paste (optional)
    - **Preparation**: Warm the mustard oil slightly and mix with garlic paste if desired. Massage onto the affected joint for 10-15 minutes.
    - **Why it Works**: Mustard oil improves blood flow and reduces stiffness, while garlic enhances anti-inflammatory effects.
    - **Pro Tip**: Perform this massage before bedtime for overnight relief.

Muscle Pain

16. **Arnica Gel**
    - **Ingredients**: Pre-made arnica gel
    - **Use**: Apply a thin layer to the sore muscle and massage gently.
    - **Why it Works**: Arnica reduces swelling, improves circulation, and relieves muscle soreness.
    - **Pro Tip**: Use after exercise or physical exertion to prevent delayed onset muscle soreness (DOMS).

17. **Magnesium Oil Spray**

- **Ingredients**: Pre-made magnesium oil spray
- **Use**: Spray directly onto the affected muscle and massage gently until absorbed.
- **Why it Works**: Magnesium relaxes muscles and reduces cramps by improving mineral balance.
- **Pro Tip**: Use before and after workouts for optimal muscle recovery.

18. **Cayenne Pepper Cream**
    - **Ingredients**: Pre-made cayenne pepper cream or 1 teaspoon of cayenne powder mixed with 2 tablespoons of coconut oil
    - **Preparation**: Mix cayenne powder with coconut oil to form a cream. Apply a small amount to the sore area.
    - **Why it Works**: Capsaicin in cayenne reduces pain signals and provides a warming sensation.
    - **Caution**: Avoid applying to broken or sensitive skin.

19. **Chamomile Compress**
    - **Ingredients**: 1 tablespoon of dried chamomile flowers, warm water, a clean cloth
    - **Preparation**: Boil chamomile flowers in water for 10 minutes. Soak the cloth in the solution, wring it out, and apply to the muscle for 15-20 minutes.
    - **Why it Works**: Chamomile relaxes muscles and reduces spasms, providing soothing relief.
    - **Pro Tip**: Drink chamomile tea alongside for additional relaxation benefits.

20. **Black Pepper Essential Oil Massage**
    - **Ingredients**: 2 drops of black pepper essential oil, 1 teaspoon of carrier oil (e.g., almond or coconut oil)
    - **Use**: Mix the oils and massage gently onto the sore muscle.
    - **Why it Works**: Black pepper improves circulation and reduces muscle tightness and soreness.
    - **Pro Tip**: Use after a warm bath for deeper relaxation and pain relief.

Back Pain

21. **Yoga Stretches (e.g., Cat-Cow Pose)**

- **Ingredients**: A yoga mat or soft surface
- **Use**: Perform the Cat-Cow pose by positioning yourself on all fours. Alternate between arching your back (Cow) and rounding it (Cat) slowly for 5-10 repetitions.
- **Why it Works**: Improves spinal flexibility, strengthens core muscles, and alleviates back tension.
- **Pro Tip**: Incorporate deep breathing to enhance the relaxing effect.

22. **Warm Water Bottle Therapy**
    - **Ingredients**: A hot water bottle or heating pad, a towel
    - **Use**: Fill the bottle with warm (not scalding) water and place it on the lower back for 15-20 minutes.
    - **Why it Works**: Heat therapy relaxes muscles and improves blood circulation, reducing pain.
    - **Pro Tip**: Use during the evening while resting to promote better sleep.

23. **Devil's Claw Capsules**
    - **Ingredients**: Pre-made Devil's Claw capsules
    - **Use**: Take one capsule daily with a meal, following product instructions.
    - **Why it Works**: Devil's Claw reduces inflammation and alleviates chronic back pain, especially lower back discomfort.
    - **Pro Tip**: Combine with regular stretching exercises for better results.

24. **Turmeric Milk**
    - **Ingredients**: 1/2 teaspoon of turmeric powder, 1 cup of warm milk
    - **Preparation**: Stir turmeric into warm milk and drink before bedtime.
    - **Why it Works**: Turmeric reduces inflammation and relaxes muscles, helping relieve back pain.
    - **Pro Tip**: Add a pinch of black pepper to improve curcumin absorption.

25. **Herbal Balm (Camphor and Eucalyptus)**
    - **Ingredients**: Pre-made herbal balm or a mix of 2 drops each of camphor and eucalyptus oils in 1 teaspoon of coconut oil

- **Use**: Massage the balm or oil mixture onto the back in gentle, circular motions.
- **Why it Works**: Camphor provides a cooling effect, while eucalyptus reduces inflammation and improves circulation.
- **Pro Tip**: Apply after a warm shower for deeper penetration into the skin.

Nerve Pain

26. **St. John's Wort Oil**

    - **Ingredients**: Pre-made St. John's Wort oil
    - **Use**: Apply a small amount to the affected area and massage gently.
    - **Why it Works**: St. John's Wort soothes nerve pain and reduces inflammation.
    - **Pro Tip**: Use consistently for at least two weeks for noticeable results.

27. **Passionflower Tea**

    - **Ingredients**: 1 teaspoon of dried passionflower, 1 cup of hot water
    - **Preparation**: Steep passionflower in hot water for 10 minutes. Strain and drink warm.
    - **Why it Works**: Passionflower calms the nervous system, helping to reduce nerve pain and associated anxiety.
    - **Pro Tip**: Drink in the evening for added relaxation and improved sleep.

28. **Cold Packs for Acute Relief**

    - **Ingredients**: An ice pack or a bag of frozen peas, a towel
    - **Use**: Wrap the ice pack in a towel and apply to the affected area for 10-15 minutes.
    - **Why it Works**: Cold therapy reduces inflammation and numbs pain from nerve irritation.
    - **Pro Tip**: Alternate with heat therapy for a more comprehensive approach.

29. **Eucalyptus Oil Massage**

    - **Ingredients**: 2 drops of eucalyptus oil, 1 teaspoon of carrier oil (e.g., almond or coconut oil)
    - **Use**: Mix the oils and massage onto the affected area in circular motions.

- **Why it Works**: Eucalyptus oil reduces inflammation and improves blood flow, easing nerve pain.
- **Pro Tip**: Inhale the aroma during the massage for additional relaxation benefits.

30. Acupuncture Therapy

- **Ingredients**: Access to a licensed acupuncture practitioner
- **Use**: Schedule regular sessions to target nerve pain and improve overall well-being.
- **Why it Works**: Acupuncture stimulates specific points to reduce pain signals and promote nerve healing.
- **Pro Tip**: Combine acupuncture with herbal remedies like passionflower tea for optimal results.

Arthritis

31. Ginger and Turmeric Tea

- **Ingredients**: 1/2 teaspoon each of grated ginger and turmeric, 1 cup of hot water
- **Preparation**: Steep ginger and turmeric in hot water for 10 minutes. Strain and drink warm.
- **Why it Works**: Ginger and turmeric reduce joint inflammation and alleviate stiffness through their anti-inflammatory properties.
- **Pro Tip**: Add a pinch of black pepper to enhance curcumin absorption from turmeric.

32. Warm Paraffin Wax Treatment

- **Ingredients**: Paraffin wax, a small heating unit, gloves or plastic wrap
- **Use**: Melt the wax in the heating unit. Dip hands or feet in the wax, let the layer cool, and repeat 2-3 times. Wrap in plastic and leave for 15 minutes.
- **Why it Works**: Heat therapy improves circulation and soothes joint pain, particularly in the hands and feet.
- **Pro Tip**: Perform this treatment in the evening for improved mobility in the morning.

33. Omega-3 Supplements

- **Ingredients**: Pre-made Omega-3 fish oil capsules
- **Use**: Take one capsule daily with a meal.

- **Why it Works**: Omega-3 fatty acids reduce inflammation and improve joint lubrication, alleviating arthritis pain.
- **Pro Tip**: Include fatty fish like salmon in your diet for additional benefits.

34. Green Tea Extract Capsules

- **Ingredients**: Pre-made green tea extract capsules
- **Use**: Take one capsule daily with water.
- **Why it Works**: Green tea's antioxidants help reduce inflammation and slow cartilage degradation in arthritis patients.
- **Pro Tip**: Pair with a cup of green tea for a double dose of antioxidants.

35. White Willow Bark Tea

- **Ingredients**: 1 teaspoon of dried white willow bark, 1 cup of hot water
- **Preparation**: Steep white willow bark in hot water for 10 minutes. Strain and drink warm.
- **Why it Works**: White willow bark contains salicin, a natural compound that reduces pain and inflammation.
- **Caution**: Avoid if allergic to aspirin or similar medications.

General Pain Relief

36. Clove Oil for Topical Application

- **Ingredients**: 2 drops of clove oil, 1 teaspoon of carrier oil (e.g., coconut or olive oil)
- **Use**: Mix the oils and massage onto the affected area.
- **Why it Works**: Clove oil contains eugenol, which has natural analgesic and anti-inflammatory properties.
- **Pro Tip**: Use sparingly, as clove oil is highly concentrated.

37. Valerian Root Capsules

- **Ingredients**: Pre-made valerian root capsules
- **Use**: Take one capsule daily, preferably in the evening.

- **Why it Works**: Valerian root relaxes muscles and reduces pain, promoting better sleep.
- **Pro Tip**: Combine with chamomile tea for enhanced relaxation.

38. Cabbage Leaf Compress

- **Ingredients**: Fresh cabbage leaves, a clean cloth
- **Preparation**: Soften cabbage leaves by rolling them or warming slightly. Place on the affected area and secure with a cloth. Leave for 20-30 minutes.
- **Why it Works**: Cabbage leaves draw out inflammation and provide mild pain relief.
- **Pro Tip**: Use chilled leaves for swelling or warmed leaves for stiffness.

39. Evening Primrose Oil

- **Ingredients**: Pre-made evening primrose oil capsules
- **Use**: Take one capsule daily with water.
- **Why it Works**: Evening primrose oil is rich in gamma-linolenic acid (GLA), which reduces inflammation and pain.
- **Pro Tip**: Pair with Omega-3 supplements for enhanced anti-inflammatory effects.

40. Massage with Sesame Oil

- **Ingredients**: 2 tablespoons of sesame oil, optional: 1 teaspoon of turmeric powder
- **Use**: Warm the sesame oil slightly and massage onto the affected area for 10-15 minutes.
- **Why it Works**: Sesame oil penetrates deeply to soothe pain, while turmeric enhances anti-inflammatory effects.
- **Pro Tip**: Perform the massage after a warm bath for better absorption.

Pain Management: Summary

This chapter provided 40 natural remedies for managing different types of pain, from headaches to arthritis. Each remedy leverages nature's healing power to reduce inflammation, promote relaxation, and improve mobility.

Key Takeaways Include:

- **Joint Pain Relief**: Remedies like **ginger and turmeric tea** and **Epsom salt baths** soothe stiffness and improve flexibility.

- **Muscle and Nerve Pain**: Solutions such as **arnica gel** and **St. John's Wort oil** offer targeted relief for sore and irritated areas.

- **General Wellness**: Incorporating supplements like **Omega-3** and **evening primrose oil** into daily routines enhances long-term pain management.

By incorporating these remedies, you can achieve effective and natural pain relief while supporting overall health and well-being.

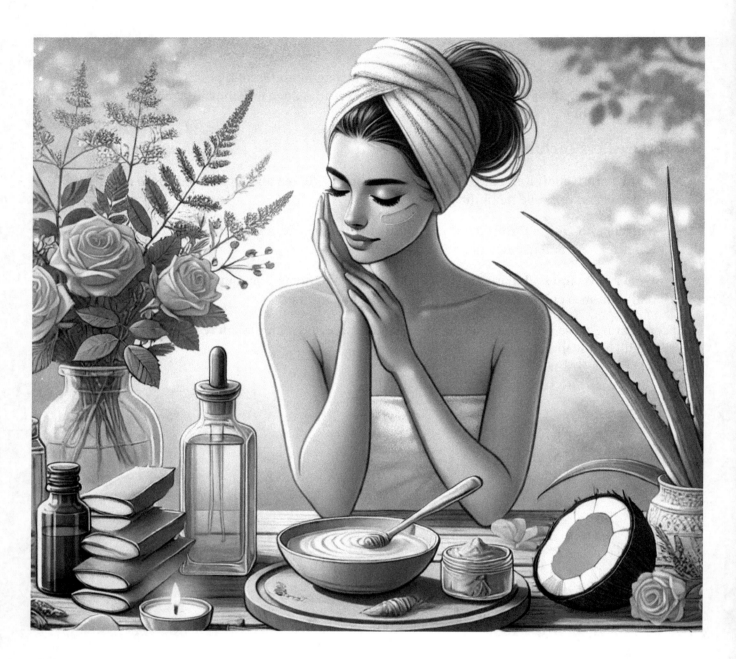

Skin and Hair Care

Introduction

Healthy skin and hair are more than just about appearance—they reflect overall well-being and self-care. Skin conditions like acne, eczema, and psoriasis, as well as hair concerns like hair loss and dandruff, can affect confidence and comfort. This chapter provides 40 natural remedies to nourish and protect your skin and hair, using time-tested ingredients and techniques.

These remedies focus on balancing hydration, reducing inflammation, and promoting natural healing, helping you achieve vibrant skin and healthy hair naturally.

Acne

1. **Tea Tree Oil (Spot Treatment)**

    - **Ingredients**: 1 drop of tea tree oil, 1 teaspoon of carrier oil (e.g., coconut or jojoba oil)
    - **Use**: Mix tea tree oil with the carrier oil and apply to acne spots using a cotton swab.
    - **Why it Works**: Tea tree oil has antimicrobial properties that reduce bacteria and inflammation.
    - **Pro Tip**: Use at night for deeper absorption and faster results.

2. **Witch Hazel Toner**

    - **Ingredients**: Pre-made witch hazel solution, cotton pads
    - **Use**: Apply witch hazel to a cotton pad and gently swipe over clean skin.
    - **Why it Works**: Witch hazel reduces excess oil and calms irritated skin.
    - **Pro Tip**: Store in the fridge for a refreshing cooling effect.

3. **Aloe Vera Gel Mask**

    - **Ingredients**: Fresh aloe vera gel or pre-made pure aloe vera gel
    - **Use**: Apply a thin layer of aloe vera gel to clean skin. Leave on for 15-20 minutes, then rinse with lukewarm water.
    - **Why it Works**: Aloe vera soothes inflammation and speeds up healing, making it ideal for acne-prone skin.
    - **Pro Tip**: Combine with a few drops of tea tree oil for added antimicrobial benefits.

4. **Green Tea Ice Cubes**

    - **Ingredients**: 1 cup of brewed green tea, ice cube tray
    - **Preparation**: Brew green tea and pour it into an ice cube tray. Freeze until solid.
    - **Use**: Rub a green tea ice cube over acne-prone areas for 1-2 minutes.
    - **Why it Works**: Green tea's antioxidants reduce redness and swelling, while the cold tightens pores.
    - **Pro Tip**: Use in the morning for a refreshing start to the day.

5. **Neem Paste**

- **Ingredients**: Fresh neem leaves or neem powder, a small amount of water
- **Preparation**: Grind neem leaves or mix neem powder with water to create a paste. Apply to acne-affected areas and leave for 15-20 minutes before rinsing.
- **Why it Works**: Neem is a natural antibacterial agent that helps reduce acne-causing bacteria and inflammation.
- **Pro Tip**: Use once or twice a week for best results.

Eczema

6. **Oatmeal Bath**
   - **Ingredients**: 1 cup of colloidal oatmeal, warm bathwater
   - **Preparation**: Add oatmeal to the bathwater and soak for 15-20 minutes.
   - **Why it Works**: Oatmeal soothes itchy and inflamed skin, providing relief for eczema symptoms.
   - **Pro Tip**: Pat skin dry gently to avoid further irritation.

7. **Calendula Cream**
   - **Ingredients**: Pre-made calendula cream or salve
   - **Use**: Apply a thin layer to affected areas as needed.
   - **Why it Works**: Calendula has anti-inflammatory and healing properties that calm eczema flare-ups.
   - **Pro Tip**: Store in a cool place for a soothing application.

8. **Coconut Oil Moisturizer**
   - **Ingredients**: Organic, cold-pressed coconut oil
   - **Use**: Apply a small amount of coconut oil to dry, eczema-affected skin.
   - **Why it Works**: Coconut oil hydrates and reduces bacterial infections on damaged skin.
   - **Pro Tip**: Use immediately after bathing to lock in moisture.

9. **Vitamin E Oil**
   - **Ingredients**: Vitamin E oil capsules or pre-made oil
   - **Use**: Pierce a capsule or use pre-made oil to apply directly to eczema patches.

- **Why it Works**: Vitamin E nourishes the skin and supports healing of damaged tissues.
- **Pro Tip**: Combine with aloe vera gel for enhanced soothing effects.

10. Chamomile Poultice

- **Ingredients**: 1 teaspoon of dried chamomile flowers, a clean cloth, hot water
- **Preparation**: Soak chamomile flowers in hot water. Strain and place the flowers in a cloth. Apply to affected areas for 10-15 minutes.
- **Why it Works**: Chamomile reduces inflammation and soothes irritated skin.
- **Pro Tip**: Use daily during eczema flare-ups for faster relief.

Psoriasis

11. Turmeric Cream

- **Ingredients**: 1 teaspoon of turmeric powder, 2 tablespoons of coconut oil
- **Preparation**: Mix turmeric powder with coconut oil to form a cream. Apply to psoriasis patches and leave for 15-20 minutes before rinsing.
- **Why it Works**: Turmeric reduces inflammation and soothes itching associated with psoriasis.
- **Pro Tip**: Use consistently to reduce flare-up frequency and severity.

12. Fish Oil Supplements

- **Ingredients**: Pre-made fish oil capsules
- **Use**: Take one capsule daily with a meal.
- **Why it Works**: Omega-3 fatty acids in fish oil reduce inflammation and promote skin healing.
- **Pro Tip**: Combine with a diet rich in fatty fish like salmon for added benefits.

13. Dead Sea Salt Bath

- **Ingredients**: 1-2 cups of Dead Sea salt, warm bathwater
- **Preparation**: Dissolve Dead Sea salt in a warm bath and soak for 15-20 minutes.
- **Why it Works**: Dead Sea salt softens scales and relieves itching, providing soothing relief for psoriasis.

- **Pro Tip**: Rinse off with clean water after the bath and apply a moisturizer to lock in hydration.

14. **Licorice Extract Gel**
    - **Ingredients**: Pre-made licorice extract gel
    - **Use**: Apply a thin layer to psoriasis patches and leave on until absorbed.
    - **Why it Works**: Licorice extract has anti-inflammatory properties that reduce redness and itching.
    - **Pro Tip**: Store in the fridge for a cooling effect during application.

15. **Aloe Vera and Vitamin D Combo**
    - **Ingredients**: 2 tablespoons of aloe vera gel, 1 vitamin D capsule
    - **Preparation**: Mix aloe vera gel with the contents of the vitamin D capsule. Apply to affected areas and leave on until absorbed.
    - **Why it Works**: Aloe vera soothes irritation, while vitamin D helps regulate skin cell production.
    - **Pro Tip**: Use daily for better management of psoriasis symptoms.

Hair Loss

16. **Rosemary Oil Scalp Massage**
    - **Ingredients**: 2 drops of rosemary essential oil, 1 teaspoon of carrier oil (e.g., coconut or jojoba oil)
    - **Use**: Mix oils and massage onto the scalp for 5-10 minutes. Leave on for an hour or overnight before washing.
    - **Why it Works**: Rosemary stimulates hair follicles, improving growth and thickness.
    - **Pro Tip**: Perform this massage 2-3 times a week for best results.

17. **Onion Juice Treatment**
    - **Ingredients**: 1 small onion, a blender, a strainer
    - **Preparation**: Blend the onion and strain to extract juice. Apply to the scalp and leave for 30 minutes before rinsing.
    - **Why it Works**: Onion juice increases blood circulation and provides sulfur to strengthen hair.

- **Pro Tip**: Add a few drops of essential oil to mask the onion smell.

18. **Castor Oil Overnight Mask**
    - **Ingredients**: 2 tablespoons of castor oil, optional: 1 teaspoon of almond oil
    - **Use**: Warm the oil slightly and apply to the scalp and hair. Leave overnight and wash off in the morning.
    - **Why it Works**: Castor oil nourishes the scalp, reduces hair fall, and promotes growth.
    - **Pro Tip**: Use a shower cap to avoid staining your pillowcase.

19. **Fenugreek Seed Paste**
    - **Ingredients**: 2 tablespoons of fenugreek seeds, water
    - **Preparation**: Soak fenugreek seeds overnight. Blend into a paste and apply to the scalp for 30 minutes before washing.
    - **Why it Works**: Fenugreek strengthens hair roots and reduces dandruff, promoting healthy growth.
    - **Pro Tip**: Rinse with cool water to enhance shine.

20. **Amla Powder Hair Pack**
    - **Ingredients**: 2 tablespoons of amla powder, 2 tablespoons of water
    - **Preparation**: Mix into a paste and apply to the scalp and hair. Leave for 30 minutes before rinsing.
    - **Why it Works**: Amla is rich in vitamin C, which strengthens hair and prevents premature greying.
    - **Pro Tip**: Combine with henna for natural conditioning.

Dandruff

21. **Apple Cider Vinegar Rinse**
    - **Ingredients**: 2 tablespoons of apple cider vinegar, 1 cup of water
    - **Use**: Mix vinegar with water and pour over your scalp after shampooing. Massage gently and rinse after 5 minutes.

- **Why it Works**: Apple cider vinegar balances scalp pH and reduces the growth of dandruff-causing fungi.
- **Pro Tip**: Use twice a week for visible results.

22. Tea Tree Shampoo

- **Ingredients**: Pre-made tea tree oil shampoo
- **Use**: Apply shampoo to wet hair, massage into the scalp, and rinse thoroughly.
- **Why it Works**: Tea tree oil's antifungal properties target dandruff at its root.
- **Pro Tip**: Let the shampoo sit on your scalp for 2-3 minutes before rinsing for maximum effectiveness.

23. Coconut Oil and Lemon Rub

- **Ingredients**: 2 tablespoons of coconut oil, 1 tablespoon of lemon juice
- **Use**: Mix coconut oil and lemon juice. Massage onto the scalp and leave for 30 minutes before rinsing.
- **Why it Works**: Coconut oil moisturizes the scalp, while lemon juice removes dandruff-causing buildup.
- **Pro Tip**: Apply weekly to maintain a healthy scalp.

24. Baking Soda Scrub

- **Ingredients**: 1 tablespoon of baking soda, 2 tablespoons of water
- **Use**: Mix into a paste and massage onto the scalp for 2-3 minutes. Rinse thoroughly.
- **Why it Works**: Baking soda exfoliates the scalp, removing dead skin and reducing flakiness.
- **Pro Tip**: Avoid overuse to prevent scalp dryness.

25. Aloe Vera and Neem Mix

- **Ingredients**: 2 tablespoons of aloe vera gel, 1 teaspoon of neem powder
- **Preparation**: Mix aloe vera gel with neem powder to form a paste. Apply to the scalp and leave for 30 minutes before rinsing.
- **Why it Works**: Aloe vera soothes irritation, and neem combats fungal infections that cause

dandruff.
- **Pro Tip**: Use as a weekly scalp treatment for ongoing maintenance.

Skin Dryness

26. **Shea Butter Balm**
    - **Ingredients**: Pre-made shea butter
    - **Use**: Apply a small amount of shea butter to dry patches and massage until absorbed.
    - **Why it Works**: Shea butter deeply hydrates and protects the skin, restoring its natural barrier.
    - **Pro Tip**: Warm the butter slightly for easier application.
    -

27. **Honey and Yogurt Mask**
    - **Ingredients**: 1 tablespoon of honey, 1 tablespoon of plain yogurt
    - **Preparation**: Mix honey and yogurt into a smooth paste. Apply to the face and leave for 15 minutes before rinsing.
    - **Why it Works**: Honey locks in moisture, while yogurt gently exfoliates and soothes dry skin.
    - **Pro Tip**: Use twice a week for consistently hydrated skin.

28. **Avocado Oil Massage**
    - **Ingredients**: 1 teaspoon of avocado oil
    - **Use**: Massage avocado oil onto dry skin in gentle, circular motions.
    - **Why it Works**: Rich in fatty acids, avocado oil nourishes and repairs dry, flaky skin.
    - **Pro Tip**: Apply before bedtime for overnight hydration.

29. **Glycerin and Rose Water Spray**
    - **Ingredients**: 1 tablespoon of glycerin, 2 tablespoons of rose water, a spray bottle
    - **Preparation**: Mix glycerin and rose water in a spray bottle. Shake well and spritz onto dry skin as needed.
    - **Why it Works**: Glycerin retains moisture, and rose water soothes and refreshes the skin.

- **Pro Tip**: Store in the fridge for a cooling effect during application.

30. **Olive Oil Moisturizer**
    - **Ingredients**: 1 teaspoon of extra virgin olive oil
    - **Use**: Massage a few drops onto dry areas and let absorb.
    - **Why it Works**: Olive oil is a natural emollient that softens and hydrates the skin.
    - **Pro Tip**: Use after a warm shower to lock in moisture.

Dark Spots

31. **Potato Juice Treatment**
    - **Ingredients**: 1 small potato, a blender, a cotton pad
    - **Preparation**: Blend the potato and strain to extract juice. Apply the juice to dark spots using a cotton pad. Leave on for 15-20 minutes, then rinse.
    - **Why it Works**: Potato juice contains enzymes and antioxidants that lighten pigmentation.
    - **Pro Tip**: Use daily for at least two weeks to see noticeable results.

32. **Lemon and Honey Mask**
    - **Ingredients**: Juice of 1/2 lemon, 1 teaspoon of honey
    - **Preparation**: Mix lemon juice with honey and apply to dark spots. Leave on for 10-15 minutes, then rinse.
    - **Why it Works**: Lemon lightens pigmentation, while honey soothes and hydrates the skin.
    - **Caution**: Avoid sunlight after application, as lemon can increase photosensitivity.

33. **Papaya Pulp Application**
    - **Ingredients**: 1/4 cup of ripe papaya pulp
    - **Use**: Apply the papaya pulp directly to dark spots and leave for 15-20 minutes. Rinse with warm water.
    - **Why it Works**: Papaya contains papain, an enzyme that exfoliates and lightens skin.
    - **Pro Tip**: Use twice a week for best results.

34. **Sandalwood Paste**

- **Ingredients**: 1 teaspoon of sandalwood powder, a few drops of rose water
- **Preparation**: Mix sandalwood powder with rose water to form a paste. Apply to dark spots and leave for 15-20 minutes. Rinse with cool water.
- **Why it Works**: Sandalwood evens out skin tone and reduces pigmentation.
- **Pro Tip**: Use during the evening for added relaxation benefits.

35. **Vitamin C Serum**

- **Ingredients**: Pre-made vitamin C serum
- **Use**: Apply a few drops of serum to dark spots after cleansing. Gently massage until absorbed.
- **Why it Works**: Vitamin C brightens skin and reduces melanin production, lightening dark spots.
- **Pro Tip**: Store in a dark, cool place to maintain potency.

Sunburn Relief

36. **Cold Milk Compress**

- **Ingredients**: 1/4 cup of cold milk, a soft cloth
- **Use**: Soak the cloth in cold milk and apply to the sunburned area for 10-15 minutes.
- **Why it Works**: Milk soothes inflamed skin and promotes healing with its natural fats and proteins.
- **Pro Tip**: Repeat several times a day for faster relief.

37. **Cucumber Gel**

- **Ingredients**: Fresh cucumber or pre-made cucumber gel
- **Preparation**: Blend cucumber into a gel-like consistency or use pre-made gel. Apply generously to sunburned areas and leave for 20 minutes before rinsing.
- **Why it Works**: Cucumber hydrates and cools irritated skin, reducing redness and swelling.
- **Pro Tip**: Store the gel in the fridge for an extra cooling effect.

38. Aloe Vera Cooling Gel

- **Ingredients**: Pure aloe vera gel
- **Use**: Apply a thick layer of aloe vera gel to the sunburned area and let it absorb.
- **Why it Works**: Aloe vera hydrates, soothes, and promotes the repair of damaged skin.
- **Pro Tip**: Reapply as needed to keep the skin hydrated.

39. Lavender Essential Oil Spray

- **Ingredients**: 5 drops of lavender essential oil, 1 cup of water, a spray bottle
- **Preparation**: Mix lavender oil with water in a spray bottle. Shake well and spritz onto sunburned skin.
- **Why it Works**: Lavender oil calms inflammation and accelerates healing.
- **Pro Tip**: Keep the spray bottle in the fridge for added cooling benefits.

40. Chamomile Infused Oil

- **Ingredients**: 1 teaspoon of dried chamomile flowers, 2 tablespoons of olive oil
- **Preparation**: Gently heat olive oil with chamomile flowers. Let cool, strain, and apply to sunburned areas.
- **Why it Works**: Chamomile reduces redness and soothes irritated skin, while olive oil provides hydration.
- **Pro Tip**: Use before bedtime to promote overnight healing.

Skin and Hair Care: Summary

This chapter provided 40 remedies to address common skin and hair concerns, promoting natural beauty and health. From acne to sunburn relief, each remedy leverages nature's power to rejuvenate and protect your skin and hair.

Key Takeaways Include:

- **Acne Management**: Solutions like **tea tree oil spot treatment** and **green tea ice cubes** target inflammation and reduce breakouts effectively.

- **Eczema and Psoriasis Relief**: Remedies such as **oatmeal baths** and **turmeric cream** soothe itchy, inflamed skin and provide lasting comfort.

- **Hair Health**: Treatments like **rosemary oil massages** and **fenugreek seed paste** strengthen hair follicles and reduce hair loss.

- **Sunburn Recovery**: Options such as **aloe vera cooling gel** and **lavender essential oil spray** offer quick relief and accelerate healing.

By incorporating these remedies into your routine, you can achieve healthy, glowing skin and strong, vibrant hair naturally. Regular use ensures sustained results and overall well-being for your skin and hair.

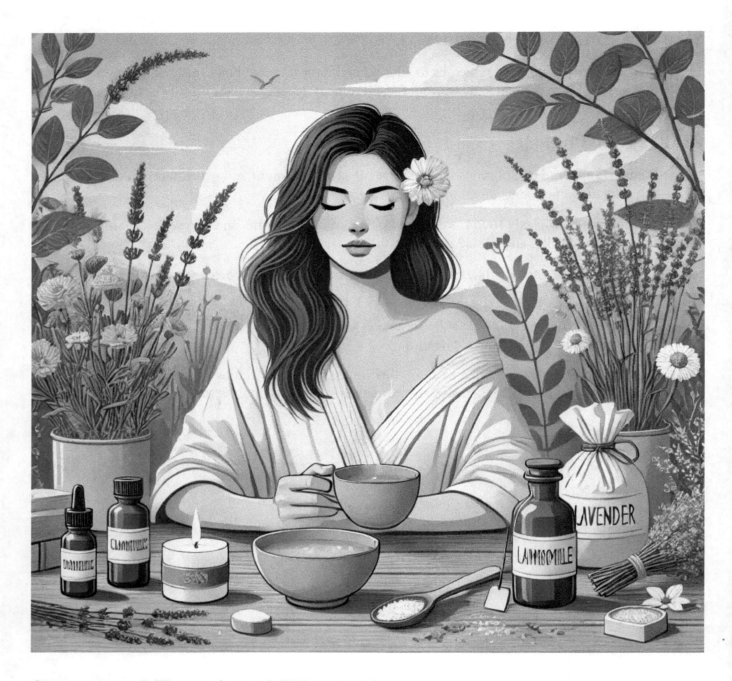

Stress and Emotional Well-Being

Introduction

Stress and emotional health are vital components of overall well-being. Prolonged anxiety, insomnia, mood swings, and burnout can take a toll on both mind and body. Thankfully, natural remedies provide holistic and effective solutions to restore balance and promote relaxation. This chapter offers 40 tried-and-true remedies for managing stress and enhancing emotional resilience.

Anxiety

1. **Lavender Tea**

    - **Ingredients**: 1 teaspoon of dried lavender flowers, 1 cup of hot water
    - **Preparation**: Steep lavender flowers in hot water for 5-7 minutes. Strain and sip slowly, savoring the aroma.
    - **Why it Works**: Lavender's calming properties reduce cortisol levels, ease nervous tension, and promote relaxation. It also enhances GABA function in the brain, which directly combats anxiety.
    - **Tip**: For enhanced benefits, combine with deep breathing exercises while drinking.

2. **Valerian Root Capsules**

    - **Ingredients**: Pre-made valerian root capsules
    - **Use**: Take one capsule during the evening or when feeling overwhelmed.
    - **Why it Works**: Valerian interacts with GABA receptors, inducing a natural calming effect without excessive drowsiness. It's especially helpful for individuals experiencing anxiety with insomnia.
    - **Caution**: Avoid combining with other sedatives to prevent over-sedation.

3. **Chamomile Tea**

    - **Ingredients**: 1 teaspoon of dried chamomile flowers, 1 cup of hot water
    - **Preparation**: Steep chamomile flowers in hot water for 5 minutes. Strain and drink warm, preferably before bed.
    - **Why it Works**: Chamomile relaxes muscles and nerves, soothing both physical and mental symptoms of anxiety.
    - **Alternative Use**: Freeze the tea into ice cubes and use as a cooling compress for stress-induced headaches.

4. **Ashwagandha Powder**

    - **Ingredients**: 1/2 teaspoon of ashwagandha powder, 1 cup of warm milk or water, a pinch of cinnamon (optional)
    - **Preparation**: Stir ashwagandha powder into the liquid, add cinnamon for flavor, and drink before bedtime.

- **Why it Works**: Ashwagandha, an adaptogen, lowers cortisol and improves long-term stress tolerance.
- **Pro Tip**: Consistent use for 4-6 weeks maximizes results.

5. **Passionflower Extract**
    - **Ingredients**: Pre-made passionflower extract
    - **Use**: Add 10-15 drops to a glass of water or tea. Sip twice daily or as needed.
    - **Why it Works**: Passionflower increases GABA levels, helping to calm overactive thoughts and reduce nervousness.
    - **Extra Tip**: Pair this remedy with journaling or meditation for a complete calming routine.

Insomnia

6. **Warm Milk with Nutmeg**
    - **Ingredients**: 1 cup of warm milk, a pinch of ground nutmeg
    - **Preparation**: Stir nutmeg into the warm milk and drink 30 minutes before bedtime.
    - **Why it Works**: Nutmeg contains myristicin, a natural sedative that promotes relaxation and induces restful sleep. The warm milk adds a comforting element, enhancing the sleep-inducing effect.
    - **Tip**: Substitute with almond or oat milk for a plant-based alternative.

7. **Lavender Pillow Spray**
    - **Ingredients**: 5 drops of lavender essential oil, 1/2 cup of water, a spray bottle
    - **Preparation**: Mix lavender oil with water in the spray bottle. Shake well and lightly mist your pillow before bedtime.
    - **Why it Works**: Lavender's aroma directly triggers the brain's relaxation centers, aiding in deeper, uninterrupted sleep.
    - **Pro Tip**: Use daily for a consistent sleep ritual.

8. **Magnesium Supplements**
    - **Ingredients**: Pre-made magnesium citrate capsules or powder
    - **Use**: Take one dose 30 minutes before bed, following product instructions.

- **Why it Works**: Magnesium relaxes muscles, regulates nervous system activity, and promotes deep, restorative sleep.
- **Extra Insight**: Regular supplementation improves overall sleep quality over time.

9. **Lemon Balm Tea**
   - **Ingredients**: 1 teaspoon of dried lemon balm leaves, 1 cup of hot water
   - **Preparation**: Steep lemon balm leaves in hot water for 7-10 minutes. Strain and drink warm.
   - **Why it Works**: Lemon balm reduces restlessness and promotes relaxation, helping you fall asleep faster.
   - **Tip**: Drink this tea while practicing slow breathing for enhanced effects.

10. **California Poppy Capsules**
    - **Ingredients**: Pre-made California poppy capsules
    - **Use**: Take one capsule before bedtime.
    - **Why it Works**: California poppy is a mild sedative that calms the nervous system and eases restlessness, making it easier to sleep.
    - **Caution**: Consult a healthcare provider if taking other sedatives.

Mood Swings

11. **St. John's Wort Capsules**
    - **Ingredients**: Pre-made St. John's Wort capsules
    - **Use**: Take one capsule daily with water.
    - **Why it Works**: St. John's Wort stabilizes mood by regulating serotonin levels, reducing irritability, and balancing emotional fluctuations.
    - **Caution**: Avoid combining with antidepressants without medical supervision.

12. **Holy Basil Tea**
    - **Ingredients**: 1 teaspoon of dried holy basil leaves, 1 cup of hot water
    - **Preparation**: Steep holy basil leaves in hot water for 5 minutes. Strain and sip slowly.
    - **Why it Works**: Holy basil balances stress hormones like cortisol, improving mood stability over

time.

- **Pro Tip**: Drink in the morning to start your day with emotional balance.

13. **Saffron Supplements**

    - **Ingredients**: Pre-made saffron capsules
    - **Use**: Take one capsule daily as per dosage instructions.
    - **Why it Works**: Saffron enhances serotonin activity in the brain, improving mood and reducing irritability.
    - **Additional Benefit**: Regular use has been linked to enhanced cognitive function.

14. **Bergamot Essential Oil Diffusion**

    - **Ingredients**: 3-4 drops of bergamot essential oil, a diffuser
    - **Preparation**: Add bergamot oil to the diffuser and let it disperse in the room for 15-20 minutes.
    - **Why it Works**: Bergamot uplifts the spirit, combats sadness, and creates a calming yet energizing environment.

15. **Yoga and Pranayama Breathing**

    - **Ingredients**: None
    - **Use**: Practice alternate nostril breathing (pranayama) for 10 minutes daily, combined with yoga poses like Child's Pose.
    - **Why it Works**: Yoga and controlled breathing regulate the autonomic nervous system, improving mood stability and reducing emotional tension.
    - **Tip**: Use during moments of emotional overwhelm to regain balance quickly.

Burnout

16. **Rhodiola Rosea Tincture**

    - **Ingredients**: Pre-made rhodiola tincture
    - **Use**: Add 10-15 drops of rhodiola tincture to a glass of water or tea. Consume once or twice daily.

- **Why it Works**: Rhodiola is an adaptogen that combats physical and mental fatigue, enhances focus, and balances cortisol levels, helping the body recover from prolonged stress.
- **Tip**: Combine this remedy with morning sunlight exposure for a powerful energy boost.

17. **Adaptogenic Herb Mixes**

    - **Ingredients**: Equal parts ashwagandha, ginseng, and holy basil powders, 1 teaspoon of honey, 1 cup of warm milk or water
    - **Preparation**: Mix the powders with honey and stir into the warm liquid. Drink in the morning for sustained energy.
    - **Why it Works**: Adaptogenic herbs work together to restore balance to the adrenal glands, combat stress, and improve endurance.
    - **Pro Tip**: Blend into a smoothie with banana for added nutrients.

18. **Aromatherapy with Rosemary**

    - **Ingredients**: 3-4 drops of rosemary essential oil, a diffuser
    - **Preparation**: Add rosemary oil to the diffuser and let the aroma fill the room for 10-15 minutes.
    - **Why it Works**: Rosemary enhances mental clarity, fights brain fog, and invigorates the senses, making it ideal for overcoming burnout.
    - **Tip**: Use during work breaks to refresh your focus.

19. **Ginseng Tea for Energy Balance**

    - **Ingredients**: 1 teaspoon of dried ginseng root, 1 cup of hot water
    - **Preparation**: Steep ginseng root in hot water for 10 minutes. Strain and drink warm.
    - **Why it Works**: Ginseng boosts stamina, improves focus, and reduces physical and mental fatigue, helping to restore energy balance.
    - **Alternative Use**: Add a slice of ginger for additional digestive support.

20. **Regular Walks in Nature**

    - **Ingredients**: Comfortable walking shoes and access to a natural environment
    - **Use**: Spend 20-30 minutes walking in a park or natural area daily or at least three times a week.

- **Why it Works**: Walking in nature lowers cortisol levels, improves mood, and revitalizes energy by connecting you to calming surroundings.
- **Pro Tip**: Leave electronic devices behind to fully immerse yourself in the experience.

Restlessness

21. Epsom Salt Foot Bath

- **Ingredients**: 1/2 cup of Epsom salt, warm water, a large basin
- **Preparation**: Dissolve Epsom salt in warm water. Soak your feet for 15-20 minutes while seated in a comfortable position.
- **Why it Works**: The magnesium in Epsom salt relaxes tense muscles and calms the nervous system, helping to reduce feelings of restlessness.
- **Tip**: Add a few drops of lavender or peppermint oil for an enhanced calming effect.

22. Peppermint Oil for Temple Massage

- **Ingredients**: 2-3 drops of peppermint essential oil, a carrier oil (e.g., coconut or almond oil)
- **Preparation**: Mix the peppermint oil with the carrier oil and gently massage onto your temples and the back of your neck. Avoid contact with eyes.
- **Why it Works**: Peppermint provides a cooling sensation that soothes tension and promotes relaxation, helping to reduce internal agitation.

23. Warm Honey Lemon Drink

- **Ingredients**: 1 teaspoon of honey, juice of half a lemon, 1 cup of warm water
- **Preparation**: Mix honey and lemon juice into the warm water and sip slowly.
- **Why it Works**: This drink soothes the throat, calms the stomach, and reduces restlessness by promoting gentle hydration and relaxation.
- **Pro Tip**: Drink before bedtime to ease the transition into sleep.

24. Acupressure on Calming Points

- **Ingredients**: None (just your hands!)
- **Use**: Apply firm but gentle pressure to the "Inner Gate" point (three finger-widths below the palm

on the inner wrist) for 2-3 minutes on each arm.

- **Why it Works**: Stimulating this point reduces nervous tension and promotes a sense of calm, helping to alleviate restlessness.

25. **Guided Meditation Apps**

- **Ingredients**: A smartphone or tablet, a meditation app (e.g., Calm, Headspace)
- **Use**: Select a meditation focused on relaxation or mindfulness. Follow along for 10-15 minutes.
- **Why it Works**: Guided meditations help focus the mind and reduce racing thoughts, providing a structured approach to managing restlessness.
- **Pro Tip**: Use noise-canceling headphones for a distraction-free experience.

Irritability

26. **Cold Shower Therapy**

- **Ingredients**: Access to a shower with cold water
- **Use**: Take a cold shower or alternate between warm and cold water for 5-7 minutes, ending with cold water.
- **Why it Works**: Cold water stimulates the vagus nerve, which helps regulate mood and reduce irritability. It refreshes both the body and mind, providing an immediate calming effect.
- **Tip**: If cold showers feel too extreme, start with lukewarm water and gradually lower the temperature over time.

27. **Tulsi Tea (Holy Basil)**

- **Ingredients**: 1 teaspoon of dried tulsi leaves, 1 cup of hot water
- **Preparation**: Steep tulsi leaves in hot water for 5 minutes. Strain and drink warm.
- **Why it Works**: Holy basil is an adaptogen that helps balance stress hormones, calm the nervous system, and reduce feelings of frustration or agitation.
- **Pro Tip**: Add a touch of honey or ginger for a soothing, flavorful twist.

28. **Cardamom-Infused Water**

- **Ingredients**: 3-4 cardamom pods, 1 liter of water

- **Preparation**: Slightly crush the cardamom pods and add them to water. Let the mixture steep for 2-3 hours or refrigerate overnight.
- **Why it Works**: Cardamom has cooling and calming properties that soothe the digestive system and relax the mind, reducing physical symptoms of irritability.

29. **Soft Music Therapy**

- **Ingredients**: A playlist of calming music or ambient sounds (e.g., classical, instrumental, or nature sounds)
- **Use**: Listen to calming music in a quiet environment for 15-20 minutes. Focus on the rhythm and melodies to relax.
- **Why it Works**: Music has been shown to reduce cortisol levels and improve mood by directly affecting the brain's emotional centers.
- **Tip**: Combine music therapy with essential oils like lavender for a multi-sensory calming effect.

30. **Rose Tea**

- **Ingredients**: 1 teaspoon of dried rose petals, 1 cup of hot water
- **Preparation**: Steep rose petals in hot water for 5-7 minutes. Strain and sip slowly.
- **Why it Works**: Rose tea has gentle mood-enhancing properties and can reduce emotional tension, making it ideal for irritability. Its aroma also helps calm the mind.

Depression

31. **Saffron and Honey Mix**

- **Ingredients**: A pinch of saffron threads, 1 teaspoon of honey
- **Preparation**: Grind saffron threads into a fine powder and mix with honey. Consume directly or dissolve in warm milk or water.
- **Why it Works**: Saffron increases serotonin levels in the brain, improving mood and alleviating symptoms of depression. Honey adds a natural energy boost and balances the blend.
- **Tip**: Consume daily for long-term emotional benefits.

32. **Regular Sunlight Exposure**

- **Ingredients**: Access to natural sunlight

- **Use**: Spend 20-30 minutes outdoors daily, preferably in the morning. Allow sunlight to touch your skin directly (face and arms).
- **Why it Works**: Sunlight stimulates vitamin D production, which plays a crucial role in regulating mood and fighting depression.

33. **Omega-3 Capsules**
    - **Ingredients**: Pre-made omega-3 fish oil capsules
    - **Use**: Take one capsule daily with a meal.
    - **Why it Works**: Omega-3 fatty acids reduce brain inflammation and enhance neurotransmitter function, improving overall emotional well-being.
    - **Caution**: Check with a doctor if taking blood-thinning medications.

34. **Journaling Practices**
    - **Ingredients**: A notebook and pen
    - **Use**: Write about your thoughts and feelings for 10-15 minutes daily. Focus on gratitude or positive events.
    - **Why it Works**: Journaling provides a healthy outlet for emotions, helps clarify thoughts, and reduces mental clutter that can exacerbate depression.

35. **Ginkgo Biloba Tea**
    - **Ingredients**: 1 teaspoon of dried ginkgo biloba leaves, 1 cup of hot water
    - **Preparation**: Steep ginkgo leaves in hot water for 10 minutes. Strain and drink warm.
    - **Why it Works**: Ginkgo improves blood flow to the brain, enhancing cognitive function and stabilizing mood.
    - **Caution**: Avoid if taking blood thinners unless approved by a healthcare provider.

General Relaxation

36. **Essential Oil Blends for Diffusion**
    - **Ingredients**: 3-4 drops of lavender essential oil, 2 drops of bergamot essential oil, a diffuser
    - **Preparation**: Add the essential oils to the diffuser with water, following the manufacturer's

instructions. Let the aroma fill the room for 20-30 minutes.

- **Why it Works**: This blend combines the calming properties of lavender with the uplifting effects of bergamot, creating a balanced and relaxing environment.
- **Tip**: Use during meditation or before bedtime for enhanced relaxation.

37. Warm Herbal Baths

- **Ingredients**: 1/2 cup of dried chamomile flowers, 1/4 cup of dried lavender, a muslin bag or cheesecloth
- **Preparation**: Place the herbs in the muslin bag and tie it securely. Add the bag to a warm bath and let it steep for 5 minutes before soaking.
- **Why it Works**: Herbal baths combine the soothing properties of heat and the calming effects of chamomile and lavender to relax tense muscles and ease the mind.
- **Pro Tip**: Play soft music or light candles to create a spa-like atmosphere.

38. Relaxation Exercises (Progressive Muscle Relaxation)

- **Ingredients**: A quiet and comfortable space
- **Use**: Lie down or sit in a comfortable position. Starting from your toes, tense each muscle group for 5 seconds, then release. Work your way up the body, finishing with the muscles in your face.
- **Why it Works**: Progressive muscle relaxation helps release built-up tension, reduces cortisol levels, and improves physical awareness, promoting overall relaxation.
- **Tip**: Combine with slow, deep breathing for maximum effect.

39. Golden Milk (Turmeric and Milk)

- **Ingredients**: 1 cup of warm milk, 1/2 teaspoon of turmeric powder, a pinch of cinnamon, honey to taste
- **Preparation**: Stir turmeric and cinnamon into the milk and heat gently. Add honey for sweetness. Drink warm, preferably in the evening.
- **Why it Works**: Turmeric reduces inflammation and promotes relaxation, while warm milk provides a comforting effect. This combination supports a calm state before sleep.
- **Alternative**: Use almond or oat milk for a plant-based version.

40. **Frankincense Incense Meditation**

- **Ingredients**: Frankincense incense sticks, an incense holder
- **Use**: Light the incense stick and place it in the holder. Sit in a comfortable position and focus on the rising smoke and its calming aroma. Meditate for 10-15 minutes.
- **Why it Works**: Frankincense reduces anxiety and promotes mindfulness, making it an excellent aid for relaxation and meditation practices.
- **Pro Tip**: Pair with guided meditations to deepen the experience.

Stress and Emotional Well-Being: Summary

The remedies in this chapter are designed to address a wide range of emotional and stress-related challenges, from anxiety and insomnia to burnout and mood swings. By integrating these natural solutions into your daily routine, you can restore balance, improve resilience, and cultivate a deeper sense of well-being.

Stress management and emotional well-being require a holistic approach that combines physical, mental, and environmental factors. While quick fixes may provide temporary relief, the remedies presented here focus on long-term benefits by addressing the root causes of stress and emotional imbalance.

Whether through the soothing power of herbal teas, the calming effects of aromatherapy, or the grounding practice of journaling, these time-tested techniques offer gentle yet effective ways to nurture your mind and body. Remember, self-care is not a luxury—it's a necessity for a vibrant and healthy life.

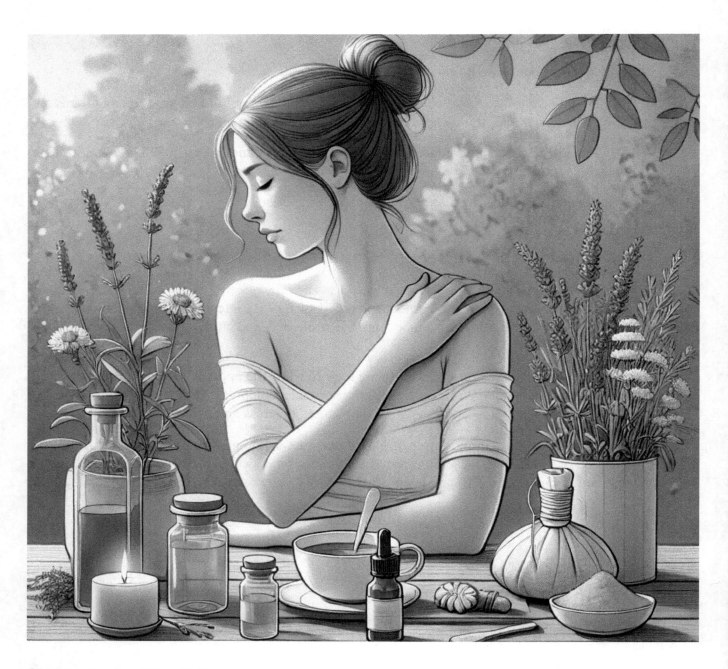

Women's Health

Introduction

Women's health presents unique challenges that range from menstrual discomfort to hormonal imbalances. Natural remedies provide effective and holistic approaches to address these needs. This chapter offers 40 remedies tailored to support women at every stage of life.

Menstrual Pain

1. **Raspberry Leaf Tea**

    - **Ingredients**: 1 teaspoon of dried raspberry leaves, 1 cup of hot water
    - **Preparation**: Steep the raspberry leaves in hot water for 10 minutes. Strain and drink warm.
    - **Why it Works**: Raspberry leaf tea is known to strengthen the uterine muscles, reducing the intensity of cramps and promoting smoother menstrual cycles.
    - **Tip**: Drink 2-3 cups daily during your period for best results.

2. **Hot Water Bottle Therapy**

    - **Ingredients**: A hot water bottle and a soft cloth
    - **Use**: Fill the hot water bottle and wrap it in a soft cloth. Place it on the lower abdomen for 15-20 minutes.
    - **Why it Works**: Heat therapy improves blood flow to the pelvic area, relaxing uterine muscles and easing menstrual cramps.
    - **Pro Tip**: Combine with a calming tea like chamomile for added relief.

3. **Ginger Tea with Honey**

    - **Ingredients**: 1 teaspoon of grated fresh ginger, 1 cup of hot water, 1 teaspoon of honey
    - **Preparation**: Steep the ginger in hot water for 10 minutes. Strain, add honey, and drink warm.
    - **Why it Works**: Ginger has anti-inflammatory properties that help alleviate pain and reduce menstrual discomfort.
    - **Tip**: Drink twice daily during heavy flow days for maximum benefit.

4. **Evening Primrose Capsules**

    - **Ingredients**: Pre-made evening primrose oil capsules
    - **Use**: Take one capsule daily, preferably with a meal.
    - **Why it Works**: Evening primrose oil contains gamma-linolenic acid (GLA), which helps regulate prostaglandins, reducing pain and inflammation.
    - **Caution**: Consult your doctor if you are on blood thinners or anticoagulants.

5. **Fennel Seed Infusion**

- **Ingredients**: 1 teaspoon of fennel seeds, 1 cup of hot water
- **Preparation**: Steep fennel seeds in hot water for 5 minutes. Strain and drink warm.
- **Why it Works**: Fennel seeds have antispasmodic properties that relax the uterine muscles, reducing cramps.
- **Tip**: Drink immediately when cramping begins for rapid relief.

PMS Symptoms

6. **Chasteberry Tincture**
   - **Ingredients**: Pre-made chasteberry tincture
   - **Use**: Add 20-30 drops to water and consume daily, preferably in the morning.
   - **Why it Works**: Chasteberry helps balance hormones by regulating the production of prolactin, easing mood swings, and reducing bloating associated with PMS.
   - **Tip**: Use consistently for at least three months to see lasting improvements.

7. **Magnesium and B6 Supplements**
   - **Ingredients**: Pre-made magnesium and B6 supplement capsules
   - **Use**: Take one capsule daily, following the dosage instructions.
   - **Why it Works**: Magnesium relaxes muscles and reduces cramps, while vitamin B6 stabilizes mood and decreases water retention during PMS.
   - **Caution**: Check with your healthcare provider if taking other medications.

8. **Black Cohosh Capsules**
   - **Ingredients**: Pre-made black cohosh capsules
   - **Use**: Take one capsule daily with water.
   - **Why it Works**: Black cohosh supports hormonal balance and alleviates PMS-related discomforts like irritability and hot flashes.
   - **Pro Tip**: Pair with a healthy diet for maximum efficacy.

9. **Peppermint Tea for Nausea**
   - **Ingredients**: 1 teaspoon of dried peppermint leaves, 1 cup of hot water

- **Preparation**: Steep peppermint leaves in hot water for 5-7 minutes. Strain and drink warm.
- **Why it Works**: Peppermint soothes the stomach and reduces bloating and nausea often associated with PMS.
- **Tip**: Keep a thermos of peppermint tea handy for quick relief.

10. **Lavender Oil Massage**

    - **Ingredients**: 3-4 drops of lavender essential oil, 1 tablespoon of carrier oil (e.g., almond or coconut oil)
    - **Preparation**: Mix lavender oil with the carrier oil and gently massage onto the lower abdomen or back in circular motions.
    - **Why it Works**: Lavender oil reduces tension, relieves pain, and promotes relaxation during PMS.
    - **Tip**: Apply after a warm bath for enhanced absorption and relaxation.

Menopause

11. **Sage Tea**

    - **Ingredients**: 1 teaspoon of dried sage leaves, 1 cup of hot water
    - **Preparation**: Steep sage leaves in hot water for 10 minutes. Strain and drink warm.
    - **Why it Works**: Sage tea helps regulate body temperature, reducing the severity of hot flashes and night sweats during menopause.
    - **Pro Tip**: Drink before bedtime to improve sleep quality and reduce nighttime discomfort.

12. **Red Clover Supplements**

    - **Ingredients**: Pre-made red clover capsules or tablets
    - **Use**: Take one capsule daily with water, following the product instructions.
    - **Why it Works**: Red clover contains phytoestrogens that mimic natural estrogen in the body, alleviating menopausal symptoms like hot flashes and mood swings.
    - **Caution**: Consult a healthcare provider before use if you have a history of hormone-sensitive conditions.

13. **Wild Yam Cream**

- **Ingredients**: Pre-made wild yam cream
- **Use**: Apply a small amount to soft areas of the skin, such as the inner arms or thighs, once or twice daily.
- **Why it Works**: Wild yam cream supports hormonal balance by providing precursors to progesterone, reducing symptoms like irritability and dryness.
- **Tip**: Use regularly for cumulative benefits over time.

14. **Maca Root Powder**
    - **Ingredients**: 1 teaspoon of maca root powder, 1 cup of warm milk or water
    - **Preparation**: Stir maca powder into the liquid and drink daily, preferably in the morning.
    - **Why it Works**: Maca root enhances energy levels, balances hormones, and alleviates symptoms like fatigue and mood swings associated with menopause.
    - **Pro Tip**: Add to smoothies for a delicious and nutritious boost.

15. **Flaxseed Smoothie**
    - **Ingredients**: 1 tablespoon of ground flaxseeds, 1 banana, 1 cup of almond milk, 1 teaspoon of honey
    - **Preparation**: Blend all ingredients until smooth. Drink immediately.
    - **Why it Works**: Flaxseeds contain lignans that help balance estrogen levels, reducing hot flashes and improving overall hormonal health.
    - **Tip**: Store flaxseeds in the refrigerator to preserve their potency.

Fertility Support

16. **Ashwagandha Root Powder**
    - **Ingredients**: 1/2 teaspoon of ashwagandha powder, 1 cup of warm milk or water
    - **Preparation**: Mix the ashwagandha powder into the liquid and drink daily, preferably in the evening.
    - **Why it Works**: Ashwagandha supports adrenal health and reduces stress, which are critical factors for improving fertility.
    - **Pro Tip**: Pair with regular yoga or meditation for maximum benefits.

17. **Shatavari Capsules**
    - **Ingredients**: Pre-made shatavari capsules
    - **Use**: Take one capsule twice daily with water, following product instructions.
    - **Why it Works**: Shatavari is a powerful adaptogen that nourishes the reproductive system and supports hormonal balance, enhancing fertility in women.

18. **Royal Jelly Supplements**
    - **Ingredients**: Pre-made royal jelly capsules or fresh royal jelly
    - **Use**: Take one capsule or a small spoonful of fresh royal jelly daily.
    - **Why it Works**: Royal jelly is rich in nutrients that improve egg quality, regulate cycles, and boost overall reproductive health.
    - **Caution**: Avoid if allergic to bees or bee products.

19. **Dong Quai Tea**
    - **Ingredients**: 1 teaspoon of dried dong quai root, 1 cup of hot water
    - **Preparation**: Steep dong quai root in hot water for 10 minutes. Strain and drink warm.
    - **Why it Works**: Dong quai enhances blood circulation to the reproductive organs and balances estrogen levels, supporting fertility.

20. **Adaptogenic Herb Mix**
    - **Ingredients**: Equal parts ashwagandha, shatavari, and maca root powders, 1 teaspoon of honey, 1 cup of warm milk or water
    - **Preparation**: Mix the powders with honey and stir into the warm liquid. Drink daily.
    - **Why it Works**: This blend combines the benefits of multiple adaptogens to optimize hormonal balance and reproductive health.
    - **Tip**: Use consistently for at least three months to see noticeable results.

PCOS Relief

21. **Spearmint Tea**
    - **Ingredients**: 1 teaspoon of dried spearmint leaves, 1 cup of hot water

- **Preparation**: Steep spearmint leaves in hot water for 5-7 minutes. Strain and drink warm.
- **Why it Works**: Spearmint tea reduces androgen levels, helping to alleviate symptoms like excessive hair growth and acne associated with PCOS.
- **Tip**: Drink 2 cups daily for consistent results.

22. Cinnamon Capsules

- **Ingredients**: Pre-made cinnamon capsules
- **Use**: Take one capsule daily with water, following product instructions.
- **Why it Works**: Cinnamon improves insulin sensitivity, reducing blood sugar levels and managing weight, which are critical in addressing PCOS symptoms.
- **Alternative Use**: Add cinnamon powder to your morning coffee or oatmeal for a dietary boost.

23. Omega-3 Fish Oil

- **Ingredients**: Pre-made omega-3 fish oil capsules
- **Use**: Take one capsule daily with a meal.
- **Why it Works**: Omega-3 fatty acids reduce inflammation and improve hormonal balance, addressing core PCOS challenges like irregular periods and elevated androgen levels.
- **Caution**: Consult a healthcare provider if on blood-thinning medications.

24. Fenugreek Seed Water

- **Ingredients**: 1 teaspoon of fenugreek seeds, 1 cup of water
- **Preparation**: Soak fenugreek seeds in water overnight. Strain and drink the infused water in the morning on an empty stomach.
- **Why it Works**: Fenugreek improves insulin sensitivity and regulates blood sugar levels, helping to manage PCOS symptoms effectively.
- **Tip**: Chew the soaked seeds for added fiber benefits.

25. Low-Glycemic Diet Support

- **Ingredients**: Foods like whole grains, legumes, green vegetables, and nuts
- **Use**: Incorporate low-glycemic foods into your meals and avoid high-sugar and refined

carbohydrates.

- **Why it Works**: A low-glycemic diet stabilizes blood sugar levels, reduces insulin resistance, and supports weight management, which are vital for PCOS relief.
- **Pro Tip**: Meal prep in advance to ensure adherence to a balanced diet.

Vaginal Health

26. **Cranberry Juice for UTI Prevention**
    - **Ingredients**: 1 cup of unsweetened cranberry juice
    - **Use**: Drink 1-2 cups daily.
    - **Why it Works**: Cranberries contain proanthocyanidins that prevent bacteria from adhering to the urinary tract walls, reducing the risk of infections.
    - **Tip**: Choose unsweetened juice to avoid added sugars that could worsen infections.

27. **Probiotic Yogurt**
    - **Ingredients**: 1 cup of plain, unsweetened probiotic yogurt
    - **Use**: Consume daily as part of a meal or snack.
    - **Why it Works**: Probiotics restore the natural vaginal flora, reducing the risk of yeast infections and maintaining a healthy pH balance.
    - **Alternative Use**: Apply topically to soothe mild irritation.

28. **Coconut Oil for Dryness Relief**
    - **Ingredients**: Organic, unrefined coconut oil
    - **Use**: Apply a small amount to the affected area as needed.
    - **Why it Works**: Coconut oil provides natural lubrication and soothes irritation caused by vaginal dryness.
    - **Caution**: Avoid use if prone to yeast infections, as oils may disrupt the natural pH balance.

29. **Calendula Tea Wash**
    - **Ingredients**: 1 teaspoon of dried calendula flowers, 1 cup of hot water

- **Preparation**: Steep calendula flowers in hot water for 10 minutes. Let it cool, then use the tea as a gentle wash.
- **Why it Works**: Calendula has antifungal and antibacterial properties, soothing irritation and promoting healing.
- **Tip**: Use as needed for external cleansing and soothing.

30. **Aloe Vera Gel**

    - **Ingredients**: Fresh aloe vera gel or pre-made organic aloe vera gel
    - **Use**: Apply a small amount externally to relieve irritation or dryness.
    - **Why it Works**: Aloe vera hydrates and soothes inflamed skin, reducing discomfort caused by dryness or mild irritation.
    - **Caution**: Ensure the gel is pure and free from additives or fragrances.

Breastfeeding Support

31. **Fenugreek Capsules**

    - **Ingredients**: Pre-made fenugreek capsules
    - **Use**: Take one capsule 2-3 times daily with water, following the product instructions.
    - **Why it Works**: Fenugreek stimulates milk production by increasing prolactin levels, helping breastfeeding mothers maintain a steady milk supply.
    - **Caution**: Consult a healthcare provider before use if you have diabetes or are taking medications for blood sugar.

32. **Blessed Thistle Tea**

    - **Ingredients**: 1 teaspoon of dried blessed thistle, 1 cup of hot water
    - **Preparation**: Steep blessed thistle in hot water for 10 minutes. Strain and drink warm, preferably 2-3 times daily.
    - **Why it Works**: Blessed thistle is known for its galactagogue properties, enhancing milk flow and supporting lactation.
    - **Tip**: Combine with fenugreek tea for a more potent lactation boost.

33. Warm Compress for Milk Flow

- **Ingredients**: A clean cloth and warm water
- **Use**: Soak the cloth in warm water, wring out the excess, and place it on the breasts for 5-10 minutes before breastfeeding.
- **Why it Works**: Warmth increases blood circulation and helps relax the milk ducts, improving milk flow and reducing engorgement.
- **Tip**: Follow with gentle massage for enhanced results.

34. Fennel Seed Infusion

- **Ingredients**: 1 teaspoon of fennel seeds, 1 cup of hot water
- **Preparation**: Steep fennel seeds in hot water for 10 minutes. Strain and drink warm.
- **Why it Works**: Fennel seeds enhance milk production while reducing colic symptoms in breastfeeding babies.
- **Pro Tip**: Drink daily for consistent benefits.

35. Oatmeal Diet

- **Ingredients**: 1 cup of cooked oats, milk or plant-based alternatives, and fruits like banana or berries
- **Use**: Incorporate oatmeal into breakfast or snacks daily.
- **Why it Works**: Oats are rich in iron and fiber, both of which support lactation and overall energy levels in breastfeeding mothers.
- **Tip**: Add flaxseeds or almond butter for an extra nutrient boost.

Hormone Balance

36. Evening Primrose Oil

- **Ingredients**: Pre-made evening primrose oil capsules
- **Use**: Take one capsule daily with a meal, following product instructions.
- **Why it Works**: Evening primrose oil contains gamma-linolenic acid (GLA), which supports hormonal balance and reduces symptoms like mood swings and breast tenderness.
- **Caution**: Consult a doctor if pregnant or breastfeeding.

37. Licorice Root Capsules

- **Ingredients**: Pre-made licorice root capsules
- **Use**: Take one capsule daily, following the dosage instructions.
- **Why it Works**: Licorice root helps regulate cortisol levels, supporting adrenal health and hormonal balance.
- **Tip**: Avoid prolonged use without consulting a healthcare provider.

38. Holy Basil Infusion

- **Ingredients**: 1 teaspoon of dried holy basil leaves, 1 cup of hot water
- **Preparation**: Steep holy basil leaves in hot water for 5 minutes. Strain and drink warm.
- **Why it Works**: Holy basil is an adaptogen that reduces cortisol, balances stress hormones, and supports overall hormonal health.
- **Pro Tip**: Drink in the morning for a refreshing start to your day.

39. Pumpkin Seed Mix

- **Ingredients**: 2 tablespoons of pumpkin seeds, 1 tablespoon of sunflower seeds, optional: chia or flaxseeds
- **Use**: Add the seed mix to smoothies, yogurt, or salads daily.
- **Why it Works**: Pumpkin seeds are rich in zinc, which supports progesterone production and overall hormonal balance.
- **Tip**: Toast the seeds lightly for added flavor and crunch.
-

40. Green Smoothies with Maca

- **Ingredients**: 1 teaspoon of maca root powder, 1 cup of spinach, 1 banana, 1 cup of almond milk, optional: honey
- **Preparation**: Blend all ingredients until smooth. Drink daily.
- **Why it Works**: Maca root helps regulate hormonal imbalances, while greens provide vital nutrients for overall endocrine health.
- **Pro Tip**: Experiment with different greens like kale or arugula for variety.

Women's Health: Summary

Women's health encompasses a variety of unique challenges and stages, from menstruation and fertility to menopause and hormonal balance. This chapter provided 40 carefully curated remedies to support women in managing these transitions and promoting overall well-being.

By using remedies like **raspberry leaf tea** for menstrual regulation, **fenugreek** for breastfeeding support, and **flaxseeds** for hormonal balance, women can address both immediate symptoms and long-term health goals naturally and effectively.

Key takeaways include:

- **Menstrual Pain**: Remedies like **ginger tea** and **hot water bottle therapy** offer quick and reliable relief.

- **Menopause Support**: Natural solutions such as **sage tea** and **red clover supplements** help reduce symptoms like hot flashes and mood swings.

- **Fertility and Hormonal Health**: Adaptogens like **ashwagandha** and nutrient-rich foods like **flaxseed smoothies** contribute to hormonal harmony and reproductive health.

The holistic approach highlighted in this chapter empowers women to take control of their health through natural remedies. While these solutions are gentle, they are powerful allies in maintaining balance and vitality. As always, consult a healthcare provider for personalized guidance, especially during pregnancy, breastfeeding, or when managing chronic conditions.

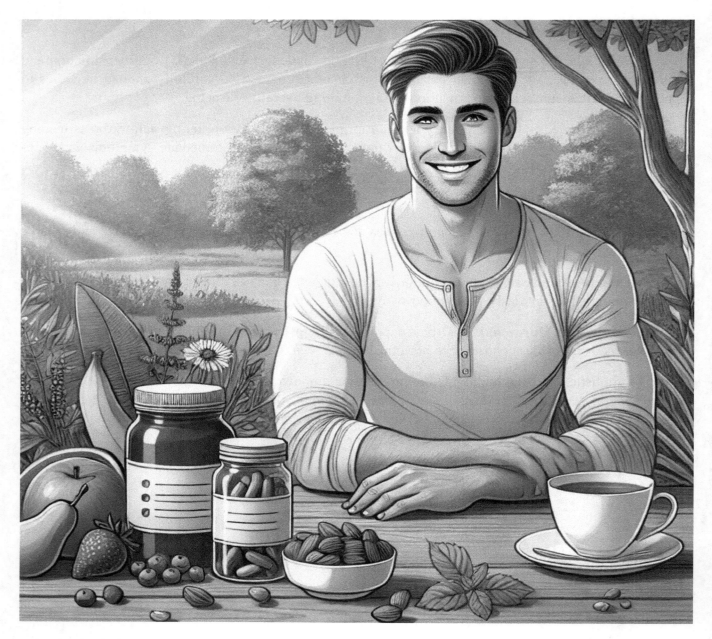

Men's Health

Introduction

Men's health encompasses a range of challenges, from maintaining prostate health to enhancing energy, stamina, and recovery. While modern medicine offers solutions, natural remedies can provide effective and sustainable support, addressing root causes rather than just symptoms. This chapter presents 40 proven remedies to help men maintain vitality, balance, and overall well-being.

Prostate Health

1. **Saw Palmetto Capsules**

    - **Ingredients**: Pre-made saw palmetto capsules
    - **Use**: Take one capsule daily with a meal, following product instructions.
    - **Why it Works**: Saw palmetto reduces inflammation and supports prostate health by inhibiting DHT (dihydrotestosterone), which contributes to prostate enlargement.
    - **Tip**: Use consistently for at least 6 weeks to see noticeable improvements.

2. **Pumpkin Seed Oil**

    - **Ingredients**: Cold-pressed pumpkin seed oil
    - **Use**: Take 1-2 teaspoons daily, or use as a salad dressing.
    - **Why it Works**: Pumpkin seed oil is rich in zinc and phytosterols, which promote prostate health and reduce urinary symptoms linked to BPH (benign prostatic hyperplasia).
    - **Pro Tip**: Combine with flaxseed oil for an even greater anti-inflammatory effect.

3. **Stinging Nettle Tea**

    - **Ingredients**: 1 teaspoon of dried stinging nettle leaves, 1 cup of hot water
    - **Preparation**: Steep nettle leaves in hot water for 5-7 minutes. Strain and drink warm.
    - **Why it Works**: Stinging nettle reduces inflammation and supports urinary flow, alleviating symptoms of an enlarged prostate.
    - **Caution**: Use gloves when handling fresh nettle leaves to avoid irritation.

4. **Lycopene-Rich Foods (Tomatoes)**

    - **Ingredients**: Fresh or cooked tomatoes, tomato juice, or tomato paste
    - **Use**: Incorporate tomatoes into daily meals, such as salads, soups, or sauces.
    - **Why it Works**: Lycopene, a powerful antioxidant, protects prostate cells from oxidative stress and reduces the risk of prostate cancer.
    - **Tip**: Cooking tomatoes with olive oil enhances lycopene absorption.

5. **Flaxseed Oil**

    - **Ingredients**: Cold-pressed flaxseed oil

- **Use**: Take 1 tablespoon daily, or add to smoothies or salads.
- **Why it Works**: Flaxseed oil is rich in omega-3 fatty acids, which reduce inflammation and promote prostate and heart health.
- **Pro Tip**: Store in the refrigerator to maintain freshness.

Stamina and Energy

6. **Ginseng Root Tea**
   - **Ingredients**: 1 teaspoon of dried ginseng root, 1 cup of hot water
   - **Preparation**: Steep ginseng root in hot water for 10 minutes. Strain and drink warm.
   - **Why it Works**: Ginseng boosts energy, enhances stamina, and reduces fatigue by improving oxygen utilization in the body.
   - **Pro Tip**: Drink in the morning for a sustained energy boost throughout the day.

7. **Beetroot Juice**
   - **Ingredients**: 1 medium beetroot, 1 cup of water
   - **Preparation**: Blend the beetroot with water, strain if desired, and drink immediately.
   - **Why it Works**: Beetroot juice increases nitric oxide levels, improving blood flow and stamina during physical activity.
   - **Tip**: Combine with apple or carrot for a sweeter flavor.

8. **Cordyceps Powder**
   - **Ingredients**: 1/2 teaspoon of cordyceps powder, 1 cup of warm water or tea
   - **Preparation**: Stir cordyceps powder into the liquid and drink daily.
   - **Why it Works**: Cordyceps enhances oxygen uptake and ATP production, improving endurance and reducing fatigue.
   - **Alternative Use**: Add to smoothies or soups for a subtle flavor boost.

9. **Ashwagandha Tincture**
   - **Ingredients**: Pre-made ashwagandha tincture
   - **Use**: Add 20-30 drops to water or tea and drink twice daily.
   - **Why it Works**: Ashwagandha is an adaptogen that reduces cortisol levels, enhancing energy and

stamina while managing stress.
- **Tip**: Use consistently for long-term benefits.

10. **Spirulina Smoothies**
    - **Ingredients**: 1 teaspoon of spirulina powder, 1 banana, 1 cup of almond milk, optional: honey
    - **Preparation**: Blend all ingredients until smooth. Drink as a morning or pre-workout boost.
    - **Why it Works**: Spirulina is rich in protein, vitamins, and minerals, providing a natural energy boost and enhancing overall vitality.
    - **Pro Tip**: Combine with greens like spinach for added nutrients.

Hair and Skin

11. **Rosemary Oil Scalp Massage**
    - **Ingredients**: 2-3 drops of rosemary essential oil, 1 tablespoon of carrier oil (e.g., coconut or jojoba oil)
    - **Use**: Mix the oils and massage gently into the scalp for 5-10 minutes. Leave on for at least an hour or overnight before washing.
    - **Why it Works**: Rosemary oil stimulates hair follicles and improves blood circulation, promoting hair growth and reducing hair loss.
    - **Pro Tip**: Use twice a week for noticeable results over time.

12. **Aloe Vera for Skin Irritation**
    - **Ingredients**: Fresh aloe vera gel or pre-made pure aloe vera gel
    - **Use**: Apply a thin layer of aloe vera gel to the affected area and leave on until absorbed. Repeat 2-3 times daily as needed.
    - **Why it Works**: Aloe vera hydrates the skin, reduces inflammation, and soothes irritation caused by sunburn, shaving, or minor rashes.
    - **Tip**: Store fresh aloe vera gel in the refrigerator for a cooling effect.

13. **Olive Oil Moisturizer**
    - **Ingredients**: 1 tablespoon of extra virgin olive oil

- **Use**: Warm the oil slightly and massage onto dry areas of the skin. Leave on overnight or rinse after 20 minutes.
- **Why it Works**: Olive oil is rich in antioxidants and healthy fats, which nourish and protect the skin, restoring moisture and elasticity.
- **Tip**: Add a drop of lavender oil for additional soothing benefits.

14. **Turmeric Capsules for Skin Health**
    - **Ingredients**: Pre-made turmeric capsules
    - **Use**: Take one capsule daily with water, following the product instructions.
    - **Why it Works**: Turmeric's anti-inflammatory and antioxidant properties combat skin conditions like acne, redness, and uneven tone.
    - **Caution**: Avoid exceeding the recommended dose to prevent gastrointestinal discomfort.

15. **Castor Oil for Beard Growth**
    - **Ingredients**: 1 teaspoon of cold-pressed castor oil
    - **Use**: Apply a small amount of castor oil to the beard area and massage thoroughly. Leave on for a few hours or overnight before washing.
    - **Why it Works**: Castor oil contains ricinoleic acid, which promotes blood flow and nourishes hair follicles, encouraging healthy beard growth.
    - **Pro Tip**: Combine with coconut oil for easier application and added hydration.

Libido Support

16. **Maca Root Powder**
    - **Ingredients**: 1 teaspoon of maca root powder, 1 cup of warm milk or water
    - **Preparation**: Mix the maca powder into the liquid and drink daily, preferably in the morning.
    - **Why it Works**: Maca root is an adaptogen that improves energy, enhances libido, and supports overall reproductive health by balancing hormones.
    - **Pro Tip**: Add to smoothies or coffee for a convenient and tasty boost.

17. **Horny Goat Weed Capsules**

- **Ingredients**: Pre-made horny goat weed capsules
- **Use**: Take one capsule daily with water, following product instructions.
- **Why it Works**: Horny goat weed contains icariin, which enhances blood flow and improves libido by supporting healthy erectile function.
- **Caution**: Consult a healthcare provider before use if you have heart conditions.

18. **Tribulus Terrestris Supplements**
    - **Ingredients**: Pre-made Tribulus terrestris capsules or tablets
    - **Use**: Take one capsule or tablet daily, following the dosage instructions.
    - **Why it Works**: Tribulus terrestris boosts testosterone production and enhances sexual performance by improving energy and stamina.
    - **Tip**: Combine with a balanced diet for maximum effectiveness.

19. **Zinc Lozenges**
    - **Ingredients**: Pre-made zinc lozenges
    - **Use**: Take one lozenge daily, following the product's dosage guidelines.
    - **Why it Works**: Zinc is essential for testosterone production and maintaining a healthy libido. It also supports immune function and overall energy.
    - **Caution**: Avoid overconsumption, as excess zinc may cause nausea or gastrointestinal discomfort.

20. **Saffron Infusion**
    - **Ingredients**: A pinch of saffron threads, 1 cup of hot water, optional: honey
    - **Preparation**: Steep saffron threads in hot water for 10 minutes. Strain and drink warm. Add honey if desired.
    - **Why it Works**: Saffron enhances mood and libido by boosting serotonin levels and improving blood flow.
    - **Pro Tip**: Use consistently for at least four weeks for noticeable effects.

Muscle Recovery

21. Whey Protein Shakes

- **Ingredients**: 1 scoop of whey protein powder, 1 cup of milk or water, optional: banana or peanut butter
- **Preparation**: Blend all ingredients until smooth. Drink immediately after a workout.
- **Why it Works**: Whey protein supports muscle repair and growth by providing essential amino acids.
- **Pro Tip**: Choose a product with minimal additives for maximum nutritional benefits.

22. Tart Cherry Juice

- **Ingredients**: 1 cup of tart cherry juice
- **Use**: Drink one cup daily, preferably after exercise or before bedtime.
- **Why it Works**: Tart cherry juice reduces muscle soreness and inflammation due to its high antioxidant and anti-inflammatory properties.
- **Tip**: Pair with magnesium-rich snacks for enhanced recovery.

23. Magnesium Spray for Sore Muscles

- **Ingredients**: Pre-made magnesium oil spray
- **Use**: Apply to sore muscles and massage gently. Allow the oil to absorb naturally.
- **Why it Works**: Magnesium relaxes muscle tension, reduces cramps, and improves overall recovery.
- **Caution**: If skin irritation occurs, dilute the spray with water.

24. Epsom Salt Baths

- **Ingredients**: 1-2 cups of Epsom salt, warm water
- **Preparation**: Dissolve Epsom salt in a warm bath and soak for 15-20 minutes.
- **Why it Works**: Epsom salt contains magnesium sulfate, which alleviates muscle soreness and promotes relaxation.
- **Pro Tip**: Add a few drops of lavender oil for a calming effect.

25. **Arnica Gel Application**

    - **Ingredients**: Pre-made arnica gel
    - **Use**: Apply a thin layer to sore or bruised areas, massaging gently. Use 2-3 times daily.
    - **Why it Works**: Arnica reduces inflammation and speeds up healing, making it ideal for minor injuries or muscle strains.
    - **Caution**: Do not apply to broken skin.

Heart Health

26. **Omega-3 Fish Oil Capsules**

    - **Ingredients**: Pre-made omega-3 fish oil capsules
    - **Use**: Take one capsule daily with a meal, following product instructions.
    - **Why it Works**: Omega-3s lower triglycerides, reduce inflammation, and promote cardiovascular health.
    - **Caution**: Consult your doctor if you're taking blood-thinning medications.

27. **Hibiscus Tea**

    - **Ingredients**: 1 teaspoon of dried hibiscus petals, 1 cup of hot water
    - **Preparation**: Steep hibiscus petals in hot water for 10 minutes. Strain and drink warm.
    - **Why it Works**: Hibiscus tea lowers blood pressure and reduces cholesterol levels, supporting heart health.
    - **Pro Tip**: Drink 1-2 cups daily for best results.

28. **Garlic Extract Tablets**

    - **Ingredients**: Pre-made garlic extract tablets
    - **Use**: Take one tablet daily with water.
    - **Why it Works**: Garlic improves circulation, lowers cholesterol, and supports healthy blood pressure.
    - **Caution**: Avoid use if you're allergic to garlic or taking anticoagulants.

29. Coenzyme Q10 Supplements

- **Ingredients**: Pre-made CoQ10 capsules or softgels
- **Use**: Take one capsule daily with a meal, following product instructions.
- **Why it Works**: CoQ10 supports heart muscle function, reduces oxidative stress, and improves energy production in cells.
- **Pro Tip**: Combine with a diet rich in fruits and vegetables for synergistic benefits.

30. Green Tea Infusion

- **Ingredients**: 1 teaspoon of green tea leaves, 1 cup of hot water
- **Preparation**: Steep green tea leaves in hot water for 2-3 minutes. Strain and drink.
- **Why it Works**: Green tea contains catechins that improve blood vessel function and lower LDL cholesterol, promoting heart health.
- **Tip**: Drink in the morning for an energy boost and antioxidant support.

Stress and Performance

31. Rhodiola Rosea Tea

- **Ingredients**: 1 teaspoon of dried Rhodiola rosea root, 1 cup of hot water
- **Preparation**: Steep rhodiola root in hot water for 10 minutes. Strain and drink warm.
- **Why it Works**: Rhodiola is an adaptogen that enhances mental focus, reduces fatigue, and improves physical performance under stress.
- **Pro Tip**: Drink in the morning for sustained energy throughout the day.

32. Adaptogen Mix for Energy Recovery

- **Ingredients**: Equal parts ashwagandha, rhodiola, and holy basil powders, 1 teaspoon of honey, 1 cup of warm milk or water
- **Preparation**: Mix the powders with honey and stir into the liquid. Drink daily.
- **Why it Works**: This blend reduces cortisol levels, improves energy recovery, and supports overall resilience to stress.
- **Tip**: Use consistently for at least 4 weeks to experience lasting benefits.

33. **Regular Cold Showers**

    - **Ingredients**: Access to a shower with cold water
    - **Use**: Take a cold shower or alternate between warm and cold water for 5-10 minutes.
    - **Why it Works**: Cold showers stimulate the vagus nerve, improving stress resilience, mental clarity, and physical endurance.
    - **Tip**: Start with lukewarm water and gradually lower the temperature.

34. **Meditation with Lavender Oil**

    - **Ingredients**: 3-4 drops of lavender essential oil, a diffuser or tissue
    - **Use**: Add lavender oil to a diffuser or dab onto a tissue. Sit in a quiet space and practice mindful breathing for 10-15 minutes.
    - **Why it Works**: Lavender reduces anxiety and promotes a calm state of mind, enhancing meditation benefits.
    - **Pro Tip**: Pair with gentle yoga for added relaxation.

35. **Regular Walks in Nature**

    - **Ingredients**: Comfortable walking shoes and access to a park or natural area
    - **Use**: Spend 20-30 minutes walking in nature daily or at least three times a week.
    - **Why it Works**: Walking in nature lowers cortisol levels, boosts mood, and improves overall mental clarity and performance.
    - **Tip**: Leave your phone behind for a distraction-free experience.

General Wellness

36. **Multivitamins with Minerals**

    - **Ingredients**: Pre-made multivitamin supplements
    - **Use**: Take one tablet daily with a meal, following product instructions.
    - **Why it Works**: Multivitamins fill nutritional gaps, supporting immune function, energy levels, and overall health.
    - **Pro Tip**: Choose a product tailored to men's health for optimal benefits.

37. Probiotic Supplements

- **Ingredients**: Pre-made probiotic capsules or tablets
- **Use**: Take one capsule daily with water, following dosage instructions.
- **Why it Works**: Probiotics maintain gut health, support digestion, and enhance the immune system.
- **Tip**: Pair with a diet rich in fermented foods for maximum results.

38. Turmeric and Ginger Tea

- **Ingredients**: 1/2 teaspoon each of turmeric and ginger powders, 1 cup of hot water, optional: honey
- **Preparation**: Mix turmeric and ginger into hot water, stir well, and add honey if desired. Drink warm.
- **Why it Works**: Turmeric and ginger reduce inflammation, boost immunity, and improve digestion, promoting overall wellness.
- **Tip**: Drink in the evening to wind down and relax.

39. Daily Bone Broth

- **Ingredients**: Pre-made bone broth or homemade broth from simmered bones and vegetables
- **Use**: Drink 1 cup of bone broth daily, preferably warm.
- **Why it Works**: Bone broth is rich in collagen, amino acids, and minerals that support joint health, skin elasticity, and immune function.
- **Pro Tip**: Add fresh herbs or garlic for added flavor and health benefits.

40. Fermented Foods

- **Ingredients**: Foods like kimchi, sauerkraut, miso, or kefir
- **Use**: Incorporate fermented foods into meals daily to promote gut health.
- **Why it Works**: Fermented foods provide probiotics and enzymes that enhance digestion, immunity, and overall well-being.
- **Tip**: Start with small portions if new to fermented foods to allow your gut to adjust.

Men's Health: Summary

This chapter provides a comprehensive guide to natural remedies for men's health, addressing critical areas like **prostate health, stamina, muscle recovery, heart health**, and overall wellness. By incorporating solutions such as **omega-3 fish oil**, **Rhodiola rosea tea**, and **probiotic supplements**, men can enhance vitality, manage stress, and maintain long-term health.

Key takeaways include:

- **Prostate Health**: Remedies like **saw palmetto capsules** and **pumpkin seed oil** offer targeted support.

- **Energy and Performance**: Adaptogens like **ashwagandha** and nutrient-rich solutions like **spirulina smoothies** boost stamina and recovery.

- **General Wellness**: Daily habits such as consuming **bone broth** and incorporating **fermented foods** support overall vitality and resilience.

As with all remedies, consult a healthcare provider to ensure the best outcomes tailored to individual needs.

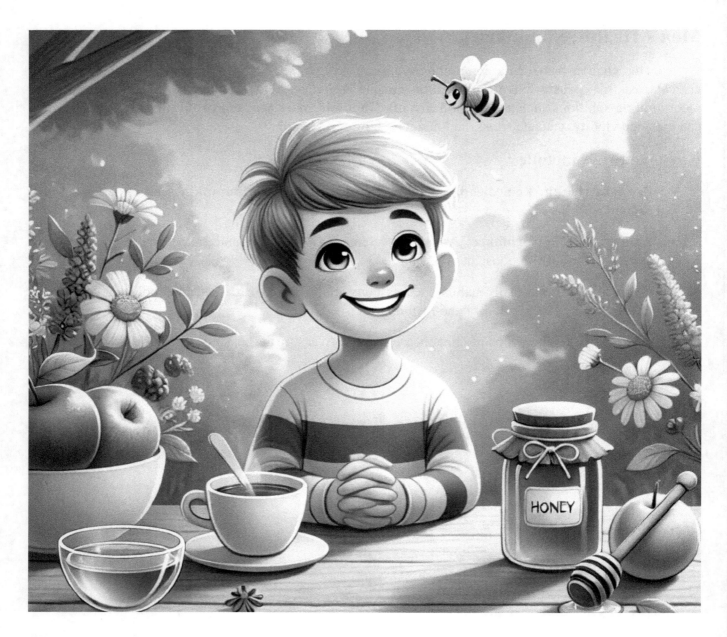

Children's Remedies

Introduction

Children's health requires gentle yet effective solutions that address common ailments without relying heavily on medications. Natural remedies provide safe, age-appropriate options for managing discomforts like teething, colic, colds, and mild fevers. These remedies harness the power of nature to soothe symptoms and support the body's natural healing processes.

This chapter focuses on 40 proven remedies tailored specifically for children's unique needs, offering solutions that are easy to prepare and safe when used under adult supervision.

Teething

1. **Chamomile Tea Compress**

    - **Ingredients**: 1 teaspoon of dried chamomile flowers, 1 cup of hot water, a soft cloth

    - **Preparation**: Steep chamomile flowers in hot water for 10 minutes. Let the tea cool to room temperature, then soak a clean cloth in the tea and gently apply it to the baby's gums.

    - **Why it Works**: Chamomile has natural anti-inflammatory and calming properties that soothe teething pain and reduce irritation.

    - **Pro Tip**: Use in the evening to help calm the baby before bedtime.

2. **Frozen Banana Teething Rings**

    - **Ingredients**: Fresh bananas, a freezer-safe tray

    - **Preparation**: Peel and slice bananas into thick rings. Place the rings on a tray and freeze for 2-3 hours. Allow the baby to gnaw on the frozen ring.

    - **Why it Works**: The cold numbs sore gums, while the banana provides a safe and tasty teething solution.

    - **Caution**: Supervise closely to prevent choking.

3. **Clove Oil Dilution for Gums**

    - **Ingredients**: 1 drop of clove essential oil, 1 tablespoon of carrier oil (e.g., coconut or olive oil)

    - **Use**: Mix clove oil with the carrier oil. Apply a small amount to your fingertip or a cotton swab and gently massage the baby's gums.

    - **Why it Works**: Clove oil contains eugenol, a natural anesthetic that relieves gum pain.

    - **Caution**: Ensure the mixture is well-diluted to avoid irritation.

4. **Silicone Teething Toys (Chilled)**

    - **Ingredients**: BPA-free silicone teething toys

    - **Use**: Chill the teething toy in the refrigerator for 20-30 minutes before giving it to the baby.

    - **Why it Works**: The cold reduces gum inflammation, while the toy provides a safe surface for chewing.

    - **Pro Tip**: Rotate several toys to keep them cool and ready for use.

5. **Breastmilk Popsicles**
    - **Ingredients**: Fresh breastmilk, popsicle molds
    - **Preparation**: Pour breastmilk into small popsicle molds and freeze until solid. Allow the baby to suck on the popsicle under supervision.
    - **Why it Works**: Breastmilk provides comfort and nutrition, while the cold soothes teething pain.
    - **Caution**: Use within 24 hours to ensure freshness.

Colic

6. **Fennel Seed Water**
    - **Ingredients**: 1/2 teaspoon of fennel seeds, 1 cup of hot water
    - **Preparation**: Steep fennel seeds in hot water for 10 minutes. Let cool, then offer 1-2 teaspoons of the water to the baby using a dropper.
    - **Why it Works**: Fennel relieves gas and reduces digestive discomfort, providing quick relief from colic.
    - **Pro Tip**: Store leftover fennel water in the refrigerator for up to 24 hours.

7. **Gripe Water (Homemade)**
    - **Ingredients**: 1/2 teaspoon each of chamomile, ginger, and fennel, 1 cup of water
    - **Preparation**: Simmer the ingredients in water for 5 minutes. Cool and strain. Offer 1 teaspoon to the baby as needed.
    - **Why it Works**: Gripe water combines soothing herbs to calm the digestive system and alleviate colic symptoms.
    - **Caution**: Use sparingly to avoid overuse.

8. **Warm Tummy Compress**
    - **Ingredients**: A clean cloth, warm water
    - **Use**: Soak the cloth in warm (not hot) water, wring out excess water, and gently place it on the baby's tummy for 5-10 minutes.
    - **Why it Works**: Warmth relaxes the abdominal muscles, reducing cramping and gas.
    - **Caution**: Always test the temperature on your wrist before applying.

9. **Bicycle Leg Exercises**

    - **Ingredients**: None

    - **Use**: Lay the baby on their back. Hold their ankles and gently move their legs in a bicycle motion for 1-2 minutes. Repeat several times daily.

    - **Why it Works**: This motion helps release trapped gas, easing colic discomfort.

    - **Pro Tip**: Combine with a warm compress for greater effectiveness.

10. **Baby Massage with Coconut Oil**

    - **Ingredients**: 1 teaspoon of organic coconut oil

    - **Use**: Warm the oil between your palms and gently massage the baby's tummy in circular motions for 5-10 minutes.

    - **Why it Works**: Massage stimulates digestion, promotes relaxation, and relieves colic-related discomfort.

    - **Caution**: Use gentle pressure and monitor the baby's reaction.

Mild Fevers

11. **Lukewarm Sponge Bath**

    - **Ingredients**: Lukewarm water, a soft sponge or cloth

    - **Use**: Soak the sponge or cloth in lukewarm water and gently dab the baby's forehead, arms, and legs. Avoid cold water as it may cause shivering.

    - **Why it Works**: Lukewarm water helps regulate body temperature and provides relief without causing discomfort.

    - **Tip**: Repeat every hour as needed until the fever subsides.

12. **Basil Tea for Fevers**

    - **Ingredients**: 1 teaspoon of fresh or dried basil leaves, 1 cup of hot water

    - **Preparation**: Steep basil leaves in hot water for 5-7 minutes. Cool and offer 1-2 teaspoons to the child.

    - **Why it Works**: Basil has antipyretic properties that naturally lower fever while boosting immunity.

    - **Pro Tip**: Add a drop of honey for children over 1 year for better taste.

13. **Cooling Compress with Peppermint**
    - **Ingredients**: 1 drop of peppermint oil, 1 cup of cool water, a soft cloth
    - **Preparation**: Mix peppermint oil with cool water. Soak the cloth, wring it out, and apply it to the child's forehead.
    - **Why it Works**: Peppermint has a cooling effect that helps bring down fever and provides comfort.
    - **Caution**: Avoid direct application of essential oils to the skin without dilution.

14. **Hydration with Coconut Water**
    - **Ingredients**: Fresh coconut water
    - **Use**: Offer small sips of coconut water throughout the day to keep the child hydrated.
    - **Why it Works**: Coconut water replenishes electrolytes lost due to fever and supports the body's recovery process.
    - **Pro Tip**: Serve chilled for a soothing effect.

15. **Apple Cider Vinegar Wipes**
    - **Ingredients**: 1 tablespoon of apple cider vinegar, 1 cup of water, a soft cloth
    - **Preparation**: Dilute apple cider vinegar in water. Soak the cloth, wring it out, and gently wipe the child's hands and feet.
    - **Why it Works**: Apple cider vinegar helps lower fever naturally by drawing heat away from the body.
    - **Caution**: Avoid using on broken or irritated skin.

Cough and Cold

16. **Honey and Lemon Syrup (Over 1 Year)**
    - **Ingredients**: 1 teaspoon of honey, 1 teaspoon of freshly squeezed lemon juice
    - **Preparation**: Mix honey and lemon juice thoroughly. Offer 1/2 teaspoon to the child 2-3 times daily.
    - **Why it Works**: Honey soothes the throat and reduces coughing, while lemon provides vitamin C

for immune support.

- **Caution**: Never give honey to children under 1 year due to the risk of botulism.

17. **Steam Inhalation with Eucalyptus (Supervised)**

    - **Ingredients**: A bowl of hot water, 1 drop of eucalyptus essential oil, a towel
    - **Preparation**: Add eucalyptus oil to hot water. Have the child sit near the bowl, cover their head with a towel, and inhale the steam for 5 minutes.
    - **Why it Works**: Steam loosens mucus, while eucalyptus opens airways and reduces congestion.
    - **Caution**: Ensure adult supervision to avoid burns.

18. **Ginger and Turmeric Milk**

    - **Ingredients**: 1/2 teaspoon each of ginger powder and turmeric powder, 1 cup of warm milk
    - **Preparation**: Mix ginger and turmeric into warm milk. Stir well and serve.
    - **Why it Works**: Ginger and turmeric have anti-inflammatory and immune-boosting properties that alleviate cold symptoms.
    - **Pro Tip**: Sweeten with honey for children over 1 year.

19. **Saline Nasal Spray**

    - **Ingredients**: Pre-made saline spray or 1 cup of water mixed with 1/4 teaspoon of salt
    - **Use**: Administer 1-2 sprays into each nostril as needed.
    - **Why it Works**: Saline spray clears nasal passages, making it easier for the child to breathe and sleep.
    - **Tip**: Use before bedtime to reduce nighttime congestion.

20. **Onion and Honey Cough Remedy**

    - **Ingredients**: 1 small onion, 2 tablespoons of honey (for children over 1 year)
    - **Preparation**: Chop the onion and mix with honey. Let it sit for 30 minutes, then strain the liquid. Offer 1 teaspoon of the liquid 2-3 times daily.
    - **Why it Works**: Onion's natural enzymes and honey's soothing properties reduce cough and support throat health.

- **Caution**: Store unused portions in the refrigerator for up to 24 hours.

Digestive Issues

21. Chamomile Tea for Stomach Upset

- **Ingredients**: 1 teaspoon of dried chamomile flowers, 1 cup of hot water
- **Preparation**: Steep chamomile flowers in hot water for 5-7 minutes. Cool and offer 1-2 teaspoons to the child.
- **Why it Works**: Chamomile calms the digestive system, reducing cramps, gas, and nausea.
- **Pro Tip**: Offer after meals to support digestion.

22. Probiotic Drops

- **Ingredients**: Pre-made probiotic drops suitable for children
- **Use**: Administer the recommended number of drops directly into the child's mouth or mixed with milk or water.
- **Why it Works**: Probiotics restore gut flora, improving digestion and alleviating issues like diarrhea and constipation.
- **Tip**: Store in the refrigerator to maintain potency.

23. Warm Water with Ginger for Gas

- **Ingredients**: 1/4 teaspoon of grated fresh ginger, 1 cup of warm water
- **Preparation**: Steep grated ginger in warm water for 5 minutes, then strain. Offer 1 teaspoon to the child.
- **Why it Works**: Ginger reduces bloating and helps release trapped gas, relieving discomfort.
- **Caution**: Ensure the water is warm, not hot, to avoid burns.

24. Banana for Diarrhea Relief

- **Ingredients**: 1 ripe banana
- **Use**: Mash the banana and serve it as a snack or mix it into plain yogurt.
- **Why it Works**: Bananas are rich in pectin, which helps firm stools and soothe the digestive system.

- **Pro Tip**: Pair with hydration to replenish lost fluids.

25. **Hydration with Electrolyte Drinks**
    - **Ingredients**: Pre-made electrolyte solution or homemade mix (1 liter of water, 1/2 teaspoon salt, 6 teaspoons sugar)
    - **Use**: Offer small sips throughout the day to keep the child hydrated.
    - **Why it Works**: Electrolyte drinks restore essential minerals and fluids lost during diarrhea or vomiting.
    - **Tip**: Add a splash of orange juice to the homemade mix for better flavor.

Skin Irritations

26. **Oatmeal Baths for Rashes**
    - **Ingredients**: 1 cup of plain oatmeal, a clean sock or muslin bag
    - **Preparation**: Place oatmeal in the sock or bag, tie securely, and soak in a tub of warm water. Let the child soak for 10-15 minutes.
    - **Why it Works**: Oatmeal soothes itching and reduces inflammation caused by rashes or eczema.
    - **Tip**: Use as needed to maintain comfort.

27. **Calendula Cream for Irritation**
    - **Ingredients**: Pre-made calendula cream
    - **Use**: Apply a small amount to the affected area 2-3 times daily.
    - **Why it Works**: Calendula has natural antibacterial and anti-inflammatory properties, promoting healing and soothing irritation.
    - **Pro Tip**: Test on a small area first to ensure no allergic reaction.

28. **Aloe Vera Gel for Mild Burns**
    - **Ingredients**: Fresh aloe vera gel or pre-made pure aloe vera gel
    - **Use**: Apply a thin layer of gel to the burned area and let it absorb naturally. Repeat 2-3 times daily.
    - **Why it Works**: Aloe vera cools the skin, reduces inflammation, and promotes healing.

- **Caution**: Avoid using on open or severe burns.

29. Coconut Oil for Dry Skin

- **Ingredients**: Organic, unrefined coconut oil
- **Use**: Warm a small amount of coconut oil between your palms and gently massage into the child's skin. Use daily or as needed.
- **Why it Works**: Coconut oil hydrates and protects the skin, reducing dryness and discomfort.
- **Pro Tip**: Apply after a bath for maximum absorption.
-

30. Cornstarch Powder for Chafing

- **Ingredients**: Pure cornstarch powder
- **Use**: Lightly dust cornstarch onto chafed areas to reduce friction and absorb moisture.
- **Why it Works**: Cornstarch keeps the skin dry and soothes irritation caused by rubbing.
- **Caution**: Avoid use near the face to prevent inhalation.

Sleep Support

31. Lavender Pillow Mist

- **Ingredients**: 2-3 drops of lavender essential oil, 1 cup of distilled water, a spray bottle
- **Preparation**: Mix lavender oil with distilled water in the spray bottle. Shake well and lightly mist the child's pillow before bedtime.
- **Why it Works**: Lavender promotes relaxation and reduces anxiety, helping the child fall asleep more easily.
- **Caution**: Ensure the mist dries completely before the child uses the pillow.

32. Bedtime Routine with Chamomile Tea

- **Ingredients**: 1 teaspoon of dried chamomile flowers, 1 cup of hot water
- **Preparation**: Steep chamomile flowers in hot water for 5 minutes, cool slightly, and offer 1-2 teaspoons to the child.
- **Why it Works**: Chamomile calms the nervous system and signals the body to prepare for sleep.

- **Pro Tip**: Pair with a calming bedtime story for a relaxing routine.

33. **Gentle Massage with Almond Oil**
    - **Ingredients**: 1 tablespoon of almond oil
    - **Use**: Warm the oil between your hands and gently massage the child's back, arms, and legs before bedtime.
    - **Why it Works**: Massage relaxes muscles, improves circulation, and promotes restful sleep.
    - **Tip**: Add a drop of lavender oil to enhance the calming effect.

34. **Warm Milk with Honey (Over 1 Year)**
    - **Ingredients**: 1 cup of warm milk, 1 teaspoon of honey
    - **Preparation**: Mix honey into warm milk and serve just before bedtime.
    - **Why it Works**: The natural sugars in honey and the warmth of the milk promote relaxation and signal sleep readiness.
    - **Caution**: Avoid for children under 1 year due to the risk of botulism.

35. **White Noise Machine**
    - **Ingredients**: A white noise machine or a smartphone app
    - **Use**: Turn on the white noise at a low volume in the child's room during bedtime.
    - **Why it Works**: White noise masks background sounds and creates a soothing environment conducive to sleep.
    - **Tip**: Experiment with different sounds (e.g., rain, ocean waves) to find the most effective one.

Immune Boosters

36. **Elderberry Syrup (Over 1 Year)**
    - **Ingredients**: Pre-made elderberry syrup or homemade (elderberries, water, honey)
    - **Use**: Offer 1/2 to 1 teaspoon daily during flu season or at the onset of cold symptoms.
    - **Why it Works**: Elderberries are rich in antioxidants and boost the immune system to fight off infections.

- **Caution**: Avoid raw elderberries as they can be toxic if not cooked properly.

37. **Vitamin C-Rich Fruits (e.g., Oranges)**
    - **Ingredients**: Fresh oranges, kiwi, or strawberries
    - **Use**: Serve as snacks or blend into smoothies.
    - **Why it Works**: Vitamin C enhances immune cell function, helping the body ward off illnesses.
    - **Pro Tip**: Combine different fruits for a nutrient-packed fruit salad.

38. **Garlic Broth for Immunity**
    - **Ingredients**: 2 garlic cloves, 2 cups of water, optional: a pinch of salt
    - **Preparation**: Simmer crushed garlic in water for 10 minutes. Strain and serve warm.
    - **Why it Works**: Garlic has antiviral and antibacterial properties that strengthen the immune system.
    - **Tip**: Serve in small sips to younger children.

39. **Probiotic Yogurt**
    - **Ingredients**: Plain, unsweetened yogurt with live cultures
    - **Use**: Serve 1-2 tablespoons as a snack or add to meals.
    - **Why it Works**: Probiotics in yogurt support gut health, which is crucial for a strong immune system.
    - **Tip**: Add a drizzle of honey for children over 1 year for flavor.

40. **Hydration with Herbal Infusions**
    - **Ingredients**: 1 teaspoon of dried peppermint or chamomile, 1 cup of hot water
    - **Preparation**: Steep the herbs in hot water for 5 minutes, cool, and offer sips to the child.
    - **Why it Works**: Herbal infusions keep the child hydrated while delivering immune-supporting benefits.
    - **Pro Tip**: Alternate between different herbal teas to keep the routine enjoyable.

Children's Remedies: Summary

This chapter provided a range of safe, natural solutions for common childhood ailments. From calming sleep routines using **lavender pillow mist** to immune-boosting remedies like **elderberry syrup**, these remedies support children's health holistically and gently.

Key takeaways include:

- **Teething and Colic Relief**: Remedies like **chamomile tea compresses** and **fennel seed water** provide effective comfort.

- **Illness Management**: Gentle options such as **lukewarm sponge baths** and **honey and lemon syrup** alleviate symptoms safely.

- **Immune Support**: Daily habits like consuming **probiotic yogurt** and **vitamin C-rich fruits** strengthen the body's defenses naturally.

As with all remedies, consult a pediatrician for guidance tailored to the child's specific needs and age.

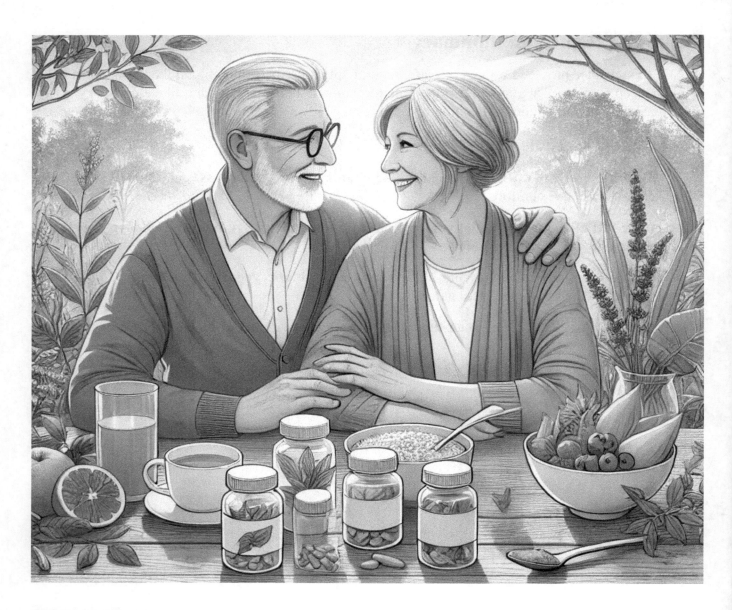

Elder Care

Introduction

Aging gracefully requires a holistic approach to health that addresses common concerns such as arthritis, memory decline, bone health, and energy support. This chapter explores 40 proven remedies designed to enhance vitality, alleviate chronic discomforts, and promote overall well-being. These natural solutions are simple to integrate into daily routines and focus on improving quality of life.

Arthritis

1. **Ginger and Turmeric Tea**

   - **Ingredients**: 1/2 teaspoon each of grated ginger and turmeric, 1 cup of hot water
   - **Preparation**: Steep ginger and turmeric in hot water for 10 minutes. Strain and drink warm.
   - **Why it Works**: Both ingredients reduce inflammation, which is key for managing arthritis symptoms.
   - **Pro Tip**: Add a pinch of black pepper to enhance curcumin absorption.

2. **Epsom Salt Foot Bath**

   - **Ingredients**: 1 cup of Epsom salt, warm water
   - **Preparation**: Dissolve Epsom salt in a basin of warm water and soak feet for 15-20 minutes.
   - **Why it Works**: Magnesium in Epsom salt relaxes muscles and reduces joint pain.
   - **Pro Tip**: Add lavender oil for relaxation and additional pain relief.

3. **Devil's Claw Capsules**

   - **Ingredients**: Pre-made Devil's Claw capsules
   - **Use**: Take one capsule daily with water, following product instructions.
   - **Why it Works**: Devil's Claw has natural anti-inflammatory properties that alleviate joint pain.
   - **Caution**: Avoid use if you have ulcers or take blood thinners.

4. **Boswellia Extract**

   - **Ingredients**: Pre-made Boswellia capsules or resin
   - **Use**: Take one capsule or chew resin daily.
   - **Why it Works**: Boswellia inhibits inflammatory enzymes, reducing joint swelling and improving mobility.
   - **Pro Tip**: Pair with turmeric capsules for enhanced results.

5. **Warm Paraffin Wax**

   - **Ingredients**: Paraffin wax, a heating device

- **Preparation**: Melt wax, cool slightly, and immerse hands or feet. Leave on for 10-15 minutes.
- **Why it Works**: The soothing heat alleviates stiffness and improves circulation.
- **Alternative Use**: Use on the neck or shoulders for broader pain relief.

Memory Support

6. **Ginkgo Biloba Capsules**
   - **Ingredients**: Pre-made Ginkgo biloba capsules
   - **Use**: Take one capsule daily with water.
   - **Why it Works**: Improves blood flow to the brain, enhancing cognitive function and memory.
   - **Pro Tip**: Combine with daily mental exercises for improved results.

7. **Rosemary Oil Diffusion**
   - **Ingredients**: 2-3 drops of rosemary oil, a diffuser
   - **Use**: Diffuse for 15-20 minutes in a quiet space.
   - **Why it Works**: Stimulates the nervous system, improving focus and mental clarity.
   - **Tip**: Inhale before mentally demanding tasks for enhanced concentration.

8. **Omega-3 Fish Oil**
   - **Ingredients**: Pre-made omega-3 capsules
   - **Use**: Take one capsule daily with a meal.
   - **Why it Works**: Supports brain health by reducing inflammation and improving neuron function.
   - **Alternative Use**: Add omega-3-rich foods like walnuts or flaxseeds to your diet.

9. **Vitamin D3 Supplements**
   - **Ingredients**: Pre-made Vitamin D3 capsules
   - **Use**: Take one capsule daily, following dosage instructions.
   - **Why it Works**: Supports cognitive health and reduces cognitive decline by improving overall immune function.
   - **Pro Tip**: Combine with outdoor walks for natural sunlight exposure.

10. **Acupressure for Cognitive Function**
    - **Use**: Press the point between the eyebrows or on the top of the head for 1-2 minutes daily.
    - **Why it Works**: Enhances blood flow to the brain, promoting relaxation and cognitive sharpness.
    - **Tip**: Use during meditation for added benefits.

Overall Vitality

11. **Ashwagandha Powder in Milk**
    - **Ingredients**: 1/2 teaspoon of ashwagandha powder, 1 cup of warm milk
    - **Preparation**: Stir the powder into the milk and drink before bedtime.
    - **Why it Works**: Reduces stress and enhances overall vitality by balancing cortisol levels.
    - **Pro Tip**: Sweeten with honey for added relaxation.

12. **Bone Broth Soup**
    - **Ingredients**: Pre-made bone broth or homemade (simmered bones with vegetables)
    - **Use**: Drink 1 cup daily.
    - **Why it Works**: Provides collagen and essential minerals for joint and skin health.
    - **Alternative Use**: Use as a base for soups or stews for added nutrition.

13. **Herbal Green Smoothies**
    - **Ingredients**: Spinach, kale, 1 banana, 1 cup of almond milk
    - **Preparation**: Blend until smooth. Drink daily.
    - **Why it Works**: Antioxidants in greens boost energy and fight oxidative stress.
    - **Pro Tip**: Rotate greens like arugula or Swiss chard for variety.

14. **Spirulina Tablets**
    - **Ingredients**: Pre-made spirulina tablets
    - **Use**: Take one tablet daily with water.
    - **Why it Works**: Spirulina provides essential nutrients that support energy and immunity.

- **Tip**: Look for certified organic products to ensure purity.

15. **Bee Pollen**
    - **Ingredients**: Raw bee pollen granules
    - **Use**: Add 1 teaspoon to smoothies or yogurt daily.
    - **Why it Works**: A nutrient powerhouse that boosts stamina and supports overall health.
    - **Caution**: Avoid if allergic to bee products.

Bone Health

16. **Calcium-Rich Foods (Sesame Seeds)**
    - **Ingredients**: Sesame seeds, almond butter, or tahini
    - **Use**: Sprinkle sesame seeds on salads, mix into smoothies, or use tahini as a spread.
    - **Why it Works**: Sesame seeds are an excellent source of calcium, which strengthens bones and reduces the risk of osteoporosis.
    - **Pro Tip**: Toast sesame seeds lightly to enhance flavor and absorption.

17. **Vitamin K2 Supplements**
    - **Ingredients**: Pre-made Vitamin K2 capsules
    - **Use**: Take one capsule daily with water, following dosage instructions.
    - **Why it Works**: Vitamin K2 supports calcium absorption into bones, improving density and strength.
    - **Alternative Use**: Incorporate K2-rich foods like natto or fermented cheese into meals.

18. **Eggshell Calcium Powder**
    - **Ingredients**: Clean, baked eggshells, a grinder
    - **Preparation**: Bake eggshells at 200°F for 10 minutes, grind into a fine powder, and store. Add 1/4 teaspoon to smoothies or yogurt.
    - **Why it Works**: Eggshells provide bioavailable calcium, supporting bone health naturally.
    - **Pro Tip**: Mix with Vitamin D supplements for maximum efficacy.

19. **Nettle Tea for Minerals**
    - **Ingredients**: 1 teaspoon of dried nettle leaves, 1 cup of hot water
    - **Preparation**: Steep nettle leaves in hot water for 10 minutes. Strain and drink warm.
    - **Why it Works**: Nettle is rich in calcium, magnesium, and other essential minerals for bone health.
    - **Tip**: Pair with honey for improved taste.

20. **Collagen Peptides**
    - **Ingredients**: Pre-made collagen peptide powder
    - **Use**: Add 1 scoop to coffee, tea, or smoothies daily.
    - **Why it Works**: Collagen supports bone matrix integrity, reducing the risk of fractures and maintaining joint health.
    - **Pro Tip**: Choose hydrolyzed collagen for better absorption.

Energy Support

21. **Maca Root Tea**
    - **Ingredients**: 1 teaspoon of maca root powder, 1 cup of hot water
    - **Preparation**: Stir maca root powder into hot water. Drink in the morning or mid-afternoon.
    - **Why it Works**: Maca root enhances energy and reduces fatigue by balancing hormones and supporting adrenal health.
    - **Pro Tip**: Add to smoothies for a nutrient-rich boost.

22. **Adaptogenic Herbs Mix**
    - **Ingredients**: Equal parts ashwagandha, rhodiola, and holy basil powders, 1 cup of warm milk or water
    - **Preparation**: Mix the powders into the liquid and drink daily.
    - **Why it Works**: Adaptogens reduce stress and enhance endurance by supporting the body's natural energy reserves.
    - **Tip**: Use consistently for at least four weeks for noticeable results.

23. **Morning Walks in Fresh Air**
    - **Ingredients**: Comfortable walking shoes, access to a safe walking area
    - **Use**: Walk for 20-30 minutes daily in a natural setting.
    - **Why it Works**: Regular walks improve cardiovascular health, boost energy, and reduce stress.
    - **Pro Tip**: Incorporate light stretches before and after for additional benefits.

24. **Holy Basil Leaf Infusion**
    - **Ingredients**: 1 teaspoon of dried holy basil leaves, 1 cup of hot water
    - **Preparation**: Steep holy basil leaves in hot water for 5-7 minutes. Strain and drink.
    - **Why it Works**: Holy basil reduces cortisol levels, promoting calm energy and resilience to stress.
    - **Pro Tip**: Drink in the evening for added relaxation benefits.

25. **Ginseng Tincture**
    - **Ingredients**: Pre-made ginseng tincture
    - **Use**: Add 20-30 drops to a glass of water or tea and drink once daily.
    - **Why it Works**: Ginseng enhances stamina and energy by improving oxygen uptake and circulation.
    - **Tip**: Use before mentally or physically demanding tasks for an immediate boost.

Heart Health

26. **Garlic Capsules**
    - **Ingredients**: Pre-made garlic capsules
    - **Use**: Take one capsule daily with a meal, following product instructions.
    - **Why it Works**: Garlic reduces cholesterol levels, improves blood circulation, and lowers blood pressure.
    - **Pro Tip**: For a natural option, include fresh garlic in daily meals.

27. **Hibiscus Tea Infusion**

- **Ingredients**: 1 teaspoon of dried hibiscus petals, 1 cup of hot water
- **Preparation**: Steep hibiscus petals in hot water for 10 minutes. Strain and drink warm.
- **Why it Works**: Hibiscus lowers blood pressure and improves heart health by reducing oxidative stress.
- **Tip**: Drink 1-2 cups daily for best results.

28. **Pomegranate Juice**

- **Ingredients**: Fresh pomegranate seeds or pre-made pomegranate juice
- **Use**: Consume 1/2 to 1 cup daily as a refreshing beverage.
- **Why it Works**: Pomegranate juice is rich in antioxidants that protect heart cells and improve blood flow.
- **Pro Tip**: Opt for 100% pure juice with no added sugars.

29. **Hawthorn Berry Capsules**

- **Ingredients**: Pre-made hawthorn berry capsules
- **Use**: Take one capsule daily with water, following product instructions.
- **Why it Works**: Hawthorn strengthens the heart muscle and improves circulation, reducing symptoms of heart disease.
- **Caution**: Consult a healthcare provider if taking heart medications.

30. **Coenzyme Q10**

- **Ingredients**: Pre-made CoQ10 capsules or softgels
- **Use**: Take one capsule daily with a meal.
- **Why it Works**: CoQ10 improves energy production in heart cells, supporting cardiovascular health and reducing fatigue.
- **Pro Tip**: Combine with a diet rich in fruits and vegetables for added benefits.

Immunity

31. **Elderberry Syrup**
    - **Ingredients**: Pre-made elderberry syrup or homemade (elderberries, water, honey)
    - **Use**: Take 1 teaspoon daily during flu season or at the onset of symptoms.
    - **Why it Works**: Elderberries boost immune function and reduce the duration of colds and flu.
    - **Caution**: Avoid raw elderberries, which can be toxic if not cooked properly.

32. **Echinacea Tea**
    - **Ingredients**: 1 teaspoon of dried echinacea flowers, 1 cup of hot water
    - **Preparation**: Steep echinacea flowers in hot water for 10 minutes. Strain and drink warm.
    - **Why it Works**: Echinacea stimulates immune cells, improving the body's ability to fight infections.
    - **Pro Tip**: Use at the first sign of illness for maximum effectiveness.

33. **Reishi Mushroom Powder**
    - **Ingredients**: 1/2 teaspoon of reishi mushroom powder, 1 cup of hot water
    - **Preparation**: Stir the powder into hot water and drink once daily.
    - **Why it Works**: Reishi mushrooms enhance immunity and reduce inflammation, supporting overall resilience.
    - **Alternative Use**: Add to soups or broths for a savory option.

34. **Lemon and Honey Drink**
    - **Ingredients**: Juice of 1/2 lemon, 1 teaspoon of honey, 1 cup of warm water
    - **Preparation**: Mix ingredients thoroughly and drink warm.
    - **Why it Works**: Lemon provides vitamin C, while honey soothes the throat and boosts immunity.
    - **Pro Tip**: Drink daily during colder months for preventive care.

35. **Probiotic Supplements**

- **Ingredients**: Pre-made probiotic capsules or tablets
- **Use**: Take one capsule daily with a meal.
- **Why it Works**: Probiotics improve gut health, which is closely linked to a strong immune system.
- **Tip**: Combine with fermented foods like yogurt for enhanced benefits.

Skin and Wound Healing

36. Calendula Ointment

- **Ingredients**: Pre-made calendula ointment
- **Use**: Apply a thin layer to cuts, scrapes, or irritated skin 2-3 times daily.
- **Why it Works**: Calendula has natural antibacterial and anti-inflammatory properties, promoting faster healing.
- **Caution**: Test on a small area to check for allergies.

37. Aloe Vera Gel for Burns

- **Ingredients**: Fresh aloe vera gel or pre-made pure aloe vera gel
- **Use**: Apply a thin layer to burns or irritated skin. Repeat 2-3 times daily as needed.
- **Why it Works**: Aloe vera cools the skin, reduces inflammation, and promotes cell regeneration.
- **Tip**: Store gel in the fridge for a soothing, cooling effect.

38. Comfrey Paste for Joint Pain

- **Ingredients**: 1 teaspoon of comfrey powder, a few drops of water
- **Preparation**: Mix into a paste and apply to the affected area. Cover with a clean cloth and leave for 30 minutes.
- **Why it Works**: Comfrey accelerates healing and reduces inflammation in joints and muscles.
- **Caution**: Avoid using on open wounds.

39. Manuka Honey for Wounds

- **Ingredients**: High-grade Manuka honey

- **Use**: Apply a small amount directly to the wound and cover with a sterile bandage. Change daily.
- **Why it Works**: Manuka honey has antibacterial properties that prevent infection and promote healing.
- **Pro Tip**: Use certified medical-grade Manuka honey for best results.

40. **Vitamin E Oil for Skin Repair**
    - **Ingredients**: Pre-made Vitamin E oil
    - **Use**: Apply directly to scars or dry skin and massage gently until absorbed.
    - **Why it Works**: Vitamin E nourishes the skin, reduces scar appearance, and promotes elasticity.
    - **Tip**: Use at bedtime for overnight repair.

Elder Care: Summary

This chapter offers comprehensive remedies for managing aging-related concerns, focusing on areas like heart health, immunity, and skin repair. From the cardiovascular benefits of **garlic capsules** to the healing power of **calendula ointment**, these natural solutions support a healthier, more vibrant lifestyle.

Key takeaways include:

- **Heart Health**: Remedies like **hibiscus tea** and **CoQ10** promote cardiovascular function.
- **Immune Boosting**: Daily habits such as consuming **elderberry syrup** and **probiotic supplements** strengthen the body's defenses.
- **Skin and Wound Healing**: Solutions like **Manuka honey** and **Vitamin E oil** offer effective skin care and repair.

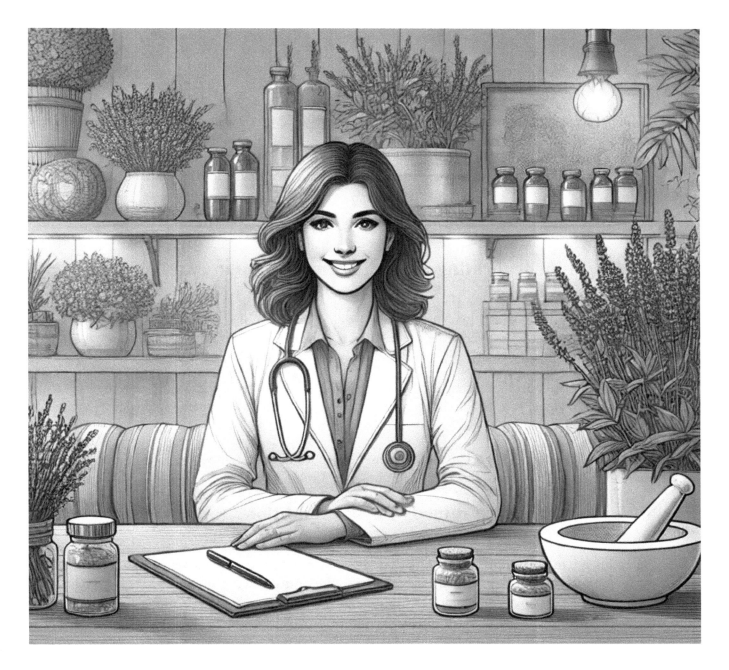

FAQs and Troubleshooting

Introduction

Natural healing offers a vast and rewarding world of remedies, but it can be daunting for beginners or even experienced practitioners to navigate. Questions arise: Which remedy is best for a particular condition? How do you ensure safety and effectiveness? What happens when a remedy doesn't work as expected?

This section addresses these challenges by providing clear answers to frequently asked questions, troubleshooting common problems, and offering practical tips for success. Whether you're new to natural remedies or looking to deepen your understanding, this guide will help you use natural healing to its fullest potential.

Understanding that natural remedies work differently from conventional medicine is key. They often target the root cause of an issue and support the body's natural ability to heal, rather than just masking symptoms. This approach requires time, patience, and a commitment to learning. With the right knowledge and preparation, natural healing can become a transformative tool for wellness.

FAQs

How do I start incorporating natural remedies into my life?

Begin by identifying one or two specific health goals. For example, if you're struggling with stress, start with simple remedies like lavender essential oil for relaxation or chamomile tea before bed. If your goal is to boost immunity, try elderberry syrup or a daily dose of vitamin C-rich foods.

Keep things manageable at first. Rather than overloading yourself with multiple remedies, focus on consistency with one or two. Gradually, as you grow more comfortable, expand your routine to include additional treatments.

Example: Someone experiencing frequent headaches might begin with peppermint oil massages, then add feverfew tea and acupressure techniques over time.

How do I choose the best remedy for my condition?

Selecting a remedy requires a combination of research, intuition, and sometimes experimentation. Start by researching the underlying cause of your condition. For instance, insomnia can stem from anxiety, hormonal imbalances, or physical discomfort. Remedies like valerian root tea (calming the mind), warm milk with nutmeg (hormonal support), or magnesium oil spray (relieving muscle tension) can be matched to the root cause.

Pro Tip: Keep a journal to track the remedies you try and their effects. This will help you identify what works best for your body.

How quickly do natural remedies work?

The timeline depends on the remedy and the condition. For acute symptoms, such as nausea or a headache, remedies like ginger tea or peppermint oil may provide relief within minutes. Chronic conditions, like arthritis or stress-induced insomnia, often require consistent use over weeks or months to yield noticeable results.

Consistency is key. Missing doses or using remedies sporadically can significantly reduce their effectiveness.

Can I combine multiple remedies?

Yes, many remedies complement each other and work synergistically. For example, pairing turmeric tea (anti-inflammatory) with a ginger compress for arthritis can address pain both internally and externally. However, avoid combining remedies with overlapping or excessive effects, such as using two strong laxatives at once.

Space remedies apart by a few hours to give your body time to process each one. For example, take adaptogenic herbs like ashwagandha in the morning for energy and chamomile tea in the evening for relaxation.

Are natural remedies safe for children and the elderly?

Generally, yes, but dosages should be adjusted, and milder remedies are often preferred. For children, remedies like chamomile tea, oatmeal baths, or honey-lemon syrup (for children over 1 year) are gentle and effective. For the elderly, remedies like bone broth, licorice root tea, or turmeric milk provide nourishment and address common issues like joint pain or digestion.

Always consult with a healthcare provider before starting new remedies for vulnerable populations.

What should I do if a remedy causes discomfort or irritation?

Discontinue the remedy immediately and assess the situation. For skin applications, rinse the area with cool water. For internal discomfort, drink plenty of water and switch to a milder alternative. Allergic reactions, though rare, can occur. Perform a patch test before applying topical remedies and start with small doses for internal ones.

If discomfort persists, consult a healthcare professional.

What happens if I don't have all the ingredients?

Many remedies have substitutions. For instance:

- If you don't have calendula for a skin treatment, aloe vera or chamomile can often serve as a substitute.
- Out of fennel seeds for digestion? Try caraway or cumin seeds instead.

Having a versatile pantry stocked with multipurpose herbs and oils, like ginger, turmeric, lavender, and coconut oil, ensures you always have options.

How do I store homemade remedies?

Proper storage is essential for maintaining potency and safety. Use dark glass containers for syrups, oils, and tinctures to protect them from light. Store creams and pastes in airtight jars in the refrigerator. Label each remedy with its preparation date and key ingredients.

Most remedies last 1-2 weeks unless otherwise specified. Discard anything that develops an off smell, color, or texture.

Why don't I see results immediately?

Natural remedies often work subtly, addressing the root cause rather than providing instant symptom relief. Chronic conditions or those resulting from long-term imbalances may require weeks of consistent use before showing noticeable improvement.

For example, while ginger tea may soothe an upset stomach immediately, adaptogens like rhodiola may take several weeks to show their effects on stress and energy.

How do I integrate remedies into a busy lifestyle?

Start small by incorporating remedies into existing habits. Drink a calming tea while working or reading. Use essential oil diffusions during your morning routine. Make larger batches of remedies, like elderberry syrup, to save time.

Pre-made options, such as capsules, tinctures, or essential oil roll-ons, can also be convenient alternatives for on-the-go use.

What if a remedy doesn't work for me?

Not all remedies work for everyone. If a remedy doesn't provide relief:

1. Reevaluate the cause of your symptoms. For example, if lavender oil isn't helping your sleep, the issue might be stress rather than insomnia, requiring an adaptogen like ashwagandha instead.
2. Experiment with alternatives. For example, if ginger tea isn't working for nausea, try peppermint tea or lemon water.

Keep an open mind and be willing to adjust your approach.

How can I tell if a remedy is of high quality?

Look for herbs that are vibrant in color and aroma, as these often indicate freshness and potency. Purchase from trusted suppliers and avoid pre-packaged blends with excessive fillers or additives. For essential oils, choose therapeutic-grade options labeled "100% pure."

Troubleshooting Common Issues

The remedy is inconvenient or time-consuming.

Solution: Simplify your process. Use pre-made tinctures or capsules when possible. Replace labor-intensive remedies with easier alternatives, such as opting for store-bought elderberry syrup instead of making your own.

The remedy isn't providing relief.

Solution: Adjust the dosage or try combining it with a complementary remedy. For instance, pair chamomile tea with a lavender-infused bath for insomnia.

Difficulty finding ingredients.

Solution: Explore online retailers specializing in herbal products or visit local farmers' markets. Substitutions, like replacing neem with tea tree oil, are also viable options.

Note

Navigating the world of natural healing requires patience, curiosity, and a willingness to adapt. By addressing these frequently asked questions and overcoming common challenges, you can unlock the full potential of natural remedies and build a sustainable path to health and well-being.

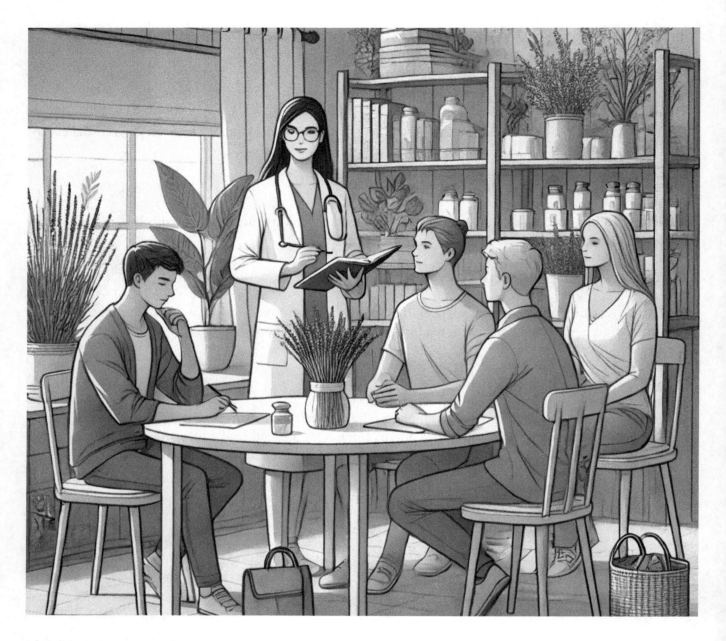

Resources and Further Reading

The journey into natural healing is a deeply personal and transformative experience. While this book offers a comprehensive guide, the world of natural remedies is vast and ever-evolving. Continuing your education and staying connected to reliable resources will empower you to deepen your practice, discover new techniques, and remain informed about the latest advancements. This chapter provides an extensive list of books, online platforms, workshops, and community networks that can serve as your roadmap to further exploration.

Books to Build a Solid Foundation

Books are timeless resources for understanding the principles and practices of natural healing. These carefully selected titles cover a range of topics, from the science behind herbs to practical applications for everyday wellness.

1. *The Green Pharmacy* by James A. Duke
   This classic guide covers hundreds of medicinal plants and their applications for various ailments. Written by a former USDA botanist, it combines scientific research with practical advice, making it an essential reference for beginners and experienced practitioners alike. The book's approachable language and indexed format make it easy to find remedies for specific conditions.

2. *Adaptogens: Herbs for Strength, Stamina, and Stress Relief* by David Winston
   Adaptogens are herbs that help the body adapt to stress and restore balance. This book offers an in-depth look at popular adaptogens like ashwagandha and rhodiola, explaining their historical uses, scientific backing, and practical applications. Perfect for those seeking to manage modern stressors naturally.

3. *Braiding Sweetgrass* by Robin Wall Kimmerer
   A poetic blend of Indigenous wisdom and scientific insight, this book explores the reciprocal relationship between humans and the natural world. While not strictly a remedy guide, it offers profound lessons on how to connect with nature and understand the spirit behind natural healing.

4. *The Herbal Medicine-Maker's Handbook* by James Green
   For those who love DIY projects, this book is a step-by-step guide to crafting herbal tinctures, salves, teas, and more. It emphasizes the joy and creativity of making remedies at home while teaching foundational skills.

5. *The Complete Book of Essential Oils and Aromatherapy* by Valerie Ann Worwood
   Essential oils are versatile tools in natural healing. This book provides detailed information on their therapeutic uses, safety guidelines, and creative ways to incorporate them into daily life. From skincare to emotional balance, this guide is comprehensive and inspiring.

Online Platforms for Continued Learning

The internet offers a wealth of resources for expanding your knowledge of natural healing. However, not all sources are reliable. Below are some trusted platforms that provide high-quality content, courses, and community support.

- **Herbal Academy**
  This online school offers courses for all skill levels, from beginner herbalism to advanced clinical practice. Topics include plant identification, herbal safety, and formulation techniques. The structured lessons, downloadable resources, and quizzes make learning engaging and effective.

- **American Botanical Council**
  A hub for research-based herbal information, this organization publishes articles, monographs, and clinical studies on medicinal plants. It's an excellent resource for those interested in the

science behind natural remedies.

- **Mountain Rose Herbs Blog**
Beyond selling herbs and oils, Mountain Rose Herbs maintains a blog filled with recipes, tutorials, and sustainability tips. It's a practical resource for those who enjoy crafting their own remedies.

- **Webinars and Online Events**
Many botanical gardens, universities, and herbal organizations host live webinars and virtual workshops on topics like growing herbs, making tinctures, and understanding herbal energetics. Search for events through platforms like Eventbrite or community herbalist groups.

Hands-On Workshops and Local Resources

Attending a workshop or joining a local community can deepen your connection to natural healing in ways that books and online resources cannot. Hands-on experiences provide the opportunity to learn from experts, practice skills, and build relationships with like-minded individuals.

- **Botanical Gardens**
Many botanical gardens offer seasonal workshops on growing, identifying, and using medicinal plants. These events often include guided tours of herb gardens, allowing participants to experience plants in their natural habitats.

- **Apothecary Classes**
Local apothecaries frequently host classes on crafting herbal remedies. These sessions might cover topics like making salves, creating custom tea blends, or using herbs for skincare.

- **Farmers' Markets and Community Centers**
Farmers' markets are often excellent places to connect with local herbalists, attend demonstrations, and purchase fresh, locally grown herbs. Community centers may also host free or low-cost classes on natural health practices.

- **Herbal Retreats**
Immersive retreats focused on natural healing offer a chance to step away from daily life and dive deeply into herbalism. These programs typically include workshops, guided nature walks, and opportunities to prepare remedies alongside experienced instructors.

Building Your Herbal Library at Home

Creating a personal library of trusted resources ensures you always have reliable information at your fingertips. Begin with a few foundational texts, then expand to include books on niche topics such as aromatherapy, adaptogens, or specific health concerns like women's wellness or immune support.

Supplement your library with digital tools. Download apps like "PlantSnap" for plant identification or "HerbList" for detailed information on herbal uses and safety. Having these resources readily available makes it easier to explore and apply natural remedies in daily life.

Engaging with Community Networks

One of the most enriching aspects of natural healing is the sense of community it fosters. Sharing knowledge, experiences, and even remedies with others creates a supportive environment for growth and learning.

- **Online Forums**
  Platforms like Reddit (e.g., r/herbalism, r/naturalremedies) and dedicated Facebook groups connect you with thousands of herbal enthusiasts. Members often share personal success stories, troubleshoot challenges, and recommend resources.

- **Local Herbalist Guilds**
  Many cities have herbalist guilds or meetup groups where members discuss topics ranging from plant identification to the ethics of wildcrafting. These gatherings provide opportunities to learn from others and share your own expertise.

- **Mentorship Opportunities**
  If you're serious about deepening your practice, consider seeking a mentor. Many experienced herbalists are open to guiding newcomers through apprenticeships or one-on-one sessions.

A Note on Sustainability and Ethics

As interest in natural remedies grows, so does the responsibility to source herbs and ingredients ethically. Overharvesting and unsustainable farming practices can endanger wild plant populations. Choose suppliers that prioritize sustainability, and whenever possible, grow your own herbs to reduce environmental impact.

- **Wildcrafting Guidelines**
  If you gather plants from the wild, follow ethical wildcrafting practices:

  - Harvest only what you need and leave plenty for regrowth.

  - Avoid endangered plants like wild ginseng unless cultivated sustainably.

  - Respect local laws and the ecosystems you're harvesting from.

- **Supporting Fair Trade**
  Purchase herbs and oils from fair-trade suppliers to ensure that the communities cultivating these resources are compensated fairly.

Closing Thoughts

The journey of natural healing is as much about personal growth as it is about health. By immersing yourself in trusted resources, connecting with communities, and engaging in hands-on learning, you can deepen your practice and share the benefits of natural remedies with others. The tools and knowledge in this chapter are just the beginning—let them inspire you to explore further and embrace the transformative power of nature.

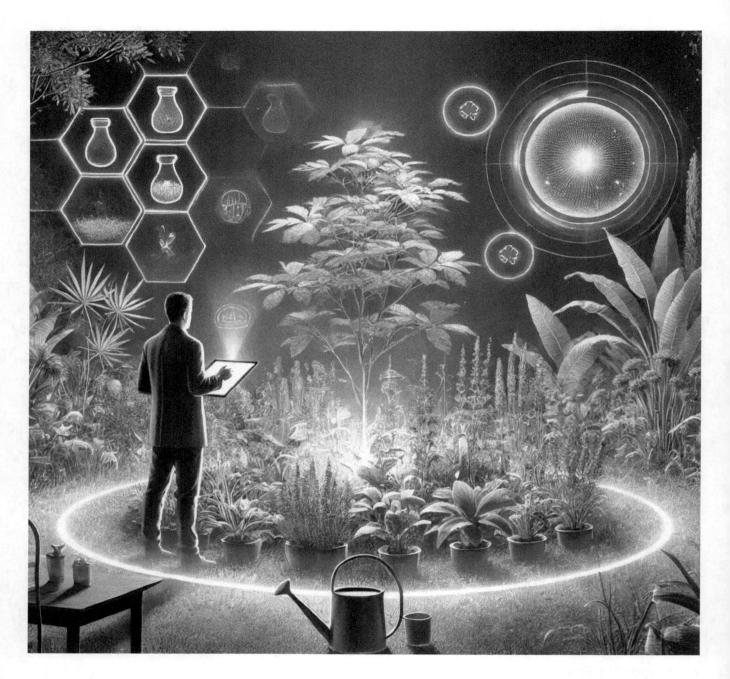

The Future of Natural Healing

The practice of natural healing is rooted in ancient traditions, yet its relevance has only grown in today's modern world. As society faces increasing challenges—ranging from chronic illnesses to environmental degradation—natural remedies offer not only a path to personal well-being but also a way to reconnect with the earth. The future of natural healing lies in harmonizing traditional wisdom with scientific innovation, making these practices more accessible, sustainable, and impactful for future generations.

Integrating Ancient Wisdom with Modern Science

For centuries, communities around the world have relied on plants, minerals, and simple practices to address health concerns. However, the scientific validation of these traditions has only recently gained momentum. Research into natural compounds like curcumin from turmeric and allicin from garlic has confirmed their powerful anti-inflammatory and antimicrobial properties, aligning with what traditional healers have known for generations.

The future promises an even deeper collaboration between traditional knowledge and cutting-edge technology. For instance:

- **Precision Herbal Medicine**: Advances in genetic testing and data analysis may lead to personalized herbal remedies tailored to an individual's unique biology. Imagine a customized adaptogenic blend designed to optimize your stress response based on your genetic markers.

- **Artificial Intelligence in Herbal Research**: AI tools are already being used to analyze historical texts and scientific studies to uncover new potential uses for plants. These insights can accelerate the discovery of remedies for complex conditions like autoimmune disorders.

Pro Tip for the Reader: While science adds credibility to natural healing, don't underestimate the value of intuition and personal experience. Combine research-backed information with your own observations to create a balanced approach.

Sustainability and Ethical Sourcing

As the popularity of natural remedies grows, so does the need to protect the ecosystems that provide these resources. Overharvesting of herbs like frankincense and wild ginseng has led to significant declines in wild populations, threatening their availability for future generations.

The future of natural healing depends on sustainable practices, such as:

- **Ethical Wildcrafting**: Collecting herbs from the wild should be done responsibly, leaving enough plants behind to ensure regrowth. For rare species, seek cultivated alternatives.

- **Supporting Regenerative Agriculture**: Herbs grown through regenerative practices not only protect the environment but also enhance soil health and biodiversity. Look for certifications like "organic" and "fair trade" when sourcing ingredients.

- **Community Gardens**: Urban and community gardens offer a way to grow medicinal plants locally, reducing the strain on wild populations.

Call to Action: As a consumer, choose suppliers that prioritize sustainability. Your purchasing decisions can have a profound impact on preserving these resources for the future.

The Role of Education in Preserving Natural Healing

Education is a cornerstone of ensuring the survival and growth of natural healing traditions. By passing down knowledge, we not only preserve cultural heritage but also empower individuals to take control of their health.

Future efforts should focus on:

- **Incorporating Herbalism into Education**: Schools and community programs can teach children and adults alike about the medicinal properties of plants, fostering a lifelong connection to nature.

- **Online Learning Platforms**: The rise of digital education allows people from all walks of life to access high-quality information about natural remedies. Courses, webinars, and virtual workshops make learning more inclusive and far-reaching.

- **Cultural Exchange**: Sharing knowledge across cultures enriches the global understanding of natural healing. For example, the use of adaptogens like ashwagandha and rhodiola in Ayurvedic and Russian traditions has gained worldwide recognition, benefiting countless individuals.

The Evolution of Natural Healing Practices

Natural healing is not static; it evolves alongside societal needs. As urbanization and fast-paced lifestyles challenge traditional practices, innovation ensures their continued relevance.

- **Convenient Formats**: Herbal remedies are increasingly available in modern, user-friendly forms, such as capsules, tinctures, and ready-to-drink teas. These innovations make it easier to incorporate remedies into daily routines.

- **Holistic Wellness Centers**: The future may see more integrative clinics where herbalists, nutritionists, and conventional doctors work together to provide comprehensive care.

- **Technology-Assisted Healing**: Mobile apps that offer reminders, dosage tracking, and guided tutorials can simplify the use of natural remedies for tech-savvy individuals.

A Vision for the Future: Imagine a world where every household has an herbal garden, every community has access to sustainable natural resources, and every individual feels empowered to take charge of their health through the wisdom of nature.

Preserving Connection to Nature

In a world increasingly dominated by technology, the practice of natural healing reminds us of our inherent connection to the earth. Beyond its physical benefits, natural healing fosters a sense of mindfulness and gratitude for the environment. Walking through a garden, preparing an herbal tea, or tending to medicinal plants offers moments of peace and reflection that modern life often lacks.

Pro Tip for the Reader: Make time for simple, grounding rituals. Whether it's brewing a cup of chamomile tea or spending a few minutes in the sun, these small acts can reconnect you with nature and its healing power.

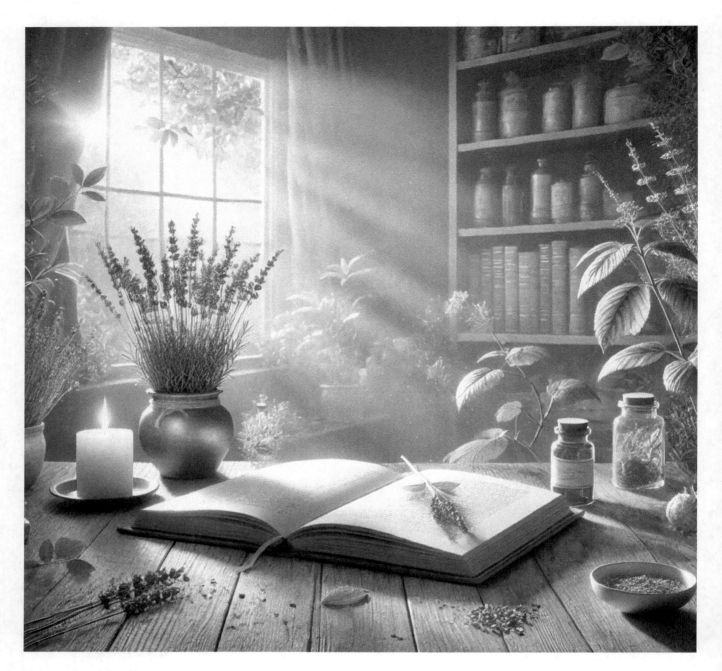

Closing Thoughts: A Message to the Reader

As you turn the final page of this book, take a moment to reflect on the journey you've undertaken. By exploring the world of natural healing, you've not only embraced a more sustainable approach to health but also reconnected with a timeless tradition that has supported humanity for centuries.

Your commitment to understanding and using natural remedies is part of a larger movement—one that values balance, resilience, and harmony with the earth. Every remedy you prepare, every plant you nurture, and every moment you spend caring for your well-being contributes to a legacy of healing that can inspire others.

Thank you for embarking on this journey. Your curiosity and dedication have not only your life but also the lives of those around you. Share what you've le continue to grow in your practice.

Remember, natural healing is not just about remedies—it's about creating a both the body and the spirit. It's about finding joy in simplicity, wisdom in nature, a knowledge that you have the tools to support your health.

From the golden fields of chamomile to the ancient forests of ginseng, nature holds endless waiting to be discovered. May this book serve as your guide, your inspiration, and your companion lifelong path of wellness and vitality.

Here's to your health, your happiness, and your connection to the healing power of nature.

Printed in the USA
CPSIA information can be obtained
at www.ICGtesting.com
LVHW081019061224
798501LV00013B/651